VEGETARIAN KIDNEY DISEASE DIET COOKBOOK

Healthy Wholesome Plant-Based Meals to Support Kidney Function

Judy Kelly

Copyright © Judy Kelly, 2024.

All rights reserved. No part of this publication may be reproduced, distributed, or transmitted in any form or by any means, including photocopying, recording, or other electronic or mechanical methods, without the prior written permission of the publisher, except in the case of brief quotations embodied in critical reviews and certain other noncommercial uses permitted by copyright law.

Table of Contents

Introduction 3
- Understanding Kidney Disease Understanding Kidney Disease 5
- The Importance of Diet in Kidney Health 7
- Why a Vegetarian Diet? 9
- Benefits of a Plant-Based Diet for Kidney Disease 12

Chapter 1: Kidney-Friendly Vegetarian Basics 15
- Key Nutrients for Kidney Health Key Nutrients for Kidney Health 15
- Foods to Include Foods to Include for Kidney Health 18
- Foods to Avoid Foods to Avoid for Kidney Health 23
- Meal Planning Tips Meal Planning Tips for Kidney Health 26

Chapter 2: Breakfast Recipes 30

Chapter 3: Lunch Recipes 40

Chapter 4: Dinner Recipes 52

Chapter 5: Snacks and Sides 65

Chapter 6: Desserts 75

Chapter 7: Drinks and Smoothies 85

Chapter 8: Supplements and Nutrition 93
- Important Supplements for Vegetarians with Kidney Disease 93
- How to Talk to Your Doctor About Supplement 95
- Managing Protein Intake 96

Chapter 9: 7-Day Meal Plan 98
- Shopping List for the Week 103

Conclusion 107

Introduction

Living with kidney disease brings unique challenges, and managing your diet is a crucial aspect of maintaining your health. Whether you've been a lifelong vegetarian or are just beginning your plant-based journey, this cookbook is designed to support you with wholesome, kidney-friendly meals that nourish both your body and soul.

For those who are new to vegetarianism, welcome to a world of vibrant, delicious foods that can make a positive difference in your health. A plant-based diet, rich in antioxidants, fiber, and essential nutrients, offers tremendous benefits, especially when managing kidney disease. For longtime vegetarians, this cookbook builds on the foundation of your existing lifestyle, offering recipes tailored to support your kidney function.

A diagnosis of kidney disease can feel overwhelming, filled with fears and uncertainties. You might worry about dietary restrictions and how they will fit into your daily life. This cookbook is here to ease those concerns, providing practical, easy-to-follow recipes that fit seamlessly into your routine. Whether you need quick breakfasts, satisfying lunches, hearty dinners, or tasty snacks, you'll find a variety of options that cater to your nutritional needs and taste preferences.

Cooking can be a therapeutic and empowering experience, especially when it involves creating meals that support your health. For new vegetarians, it's an opportunity to explore new flavors and ingredients, discovering the richness of plant-based eating. For seasoned vegetarians, it's a chance to refine and enhance your diet to better support your kidney health.

I understand the emotional and physical toll that kidney disease can take, and my goal is to offer you comfort and support through these recipes. Each dish is thoughtfully crafted to provide the nutrients essential for kidney health while being delicious and satisfying. Embracing a vegetarian diet is not just about avoiding certain foods; it's about celebrating the abundance of flavors, colors, and textures that plants offer.

Thank you for allowing me to be a part of your journey towards better health. My hope is that this cookbook becomes a trusted companion in your kitchen, offering inspiration, support, and delicious meals that make you feel good inside and out. Remember, every small step you take towards a healthier diet is a step towards a stronger, more vibrant you.

- Understanding Kidney Disease Understanding Kidney Disease

Kidney disease, also known as chronic kidney disease (CKD), is a condition where the kidneys gradually lose their ability to filter waste and excess fluids from the blood. This progressive loss of function can lead to a buildup of harmful substances in the body, affecting overall health and well-being. Understanding the basics of kidney disease can help you make informed decisions about your diet and lifestyle, which are crucial for managing this condition effectively.

The Role of the Kidneys

The kidneys are two bean-shaped organs located on either side of your spine, just below the rib cage. Their primary functions include:
- Filtering Waste and Excess Fluids: The kidneys remove waste products and excess fluids from the blood, which are then excreted as urine.
- Balancing Electrolytes: They help maintain the balance of essential minerals, such as sodium, potassium, and phosphorus, in the blood.
- Regulating Blood Pressure: The kidneys produce hormones that regulate blood pressure and control the production of red blood cells.
- Supporting Bone Health: They help activate vitamin D, which is crucial for calcium absorption and bone health.

Causes of Kidney Disease

Kidney disease can be caused by a variety of factors, including:
- Diabetes: High blood sugar levels can damage the blood vessels in the kidneys, leading to reduced function.
- High Blood Pressure: Hypertension can cause damage to the small blood vessels in the kidneys, impairing their ability to filter blood effectively.
- Glomerulonephritis: Inflammation of the kidney's filtering units can lead to chronic kidney damage.
- Polycystic Kidney Disease: A genetic disorder characterized by the growth of cysts in the kidneys.
- Recurrent Kidney Infections: Frequent infections can cause damage and scarring to the kidneys.

Symptoms of Kidney Disease
In the early stages, kidney disease often has no noticeable symptoms. As the condition progresses, symptoms may include:
- Fatigue and weakness
- Swelling in the legs, ankles, and feet
- Shortness of breath
- Nausea and vomiting
- Changes in urination patterns
- Muscle cramps and twitches
- Itchy skin and dry skin

The Importance of Diet in Kidney Health
Diet plays a vital role in managing kidney disease. By making the right food choices, you can help reduce the workload on your kidneys, maintain electrolyte balance, and prevent further damage. A kidney-friendly diet typically involves:
- Reducing Sodium Intake: To prevent fluid retention and high blood pressure.
- Limiting Potassium and Phosphorus: To avoid imbalances that can lead to heart problems and bone disease.
- Managing Protein Intake: To reduce the amount of waste the kidneys need to filter.
- Staying Hydrated: To help the kidneys function efficiently without overworking them.

Why a Vegetarian Diet?
A vegetarian diet can be particularly beneficial for individuals with kidney disease. Plant-based diets are naturally lower in saturated fats and cholesterol, which supports heart health—a crucial aspect since cardiovascular disease is a common complication of kidney disease. Additionally, vegetarian diets are rich in fruits, vegetables, and whole grains, providing essential nutrients while being easier on the kidneys.

This cookbook is designed to help you navigate your dietary needs with compassion and understanding. The recipes within offer a variety of delicious, kidney-friendly vegetarian meals that nourish your body and support your kidney function. Whether you're a long-time vegetarian or new to this way of eating, you'll find practical, enjoyable recipes that fit seamlessly into your life.

Remember, managing kidney disease is a journey, and every positive change you make brings you closer to better health and well-being.

- The Importance of Diet in Kidney Health

Diet is a cornerstone in the management and prevention of kidney disease. The foods we eat directly impact the health and function of our kidneys, and making mindful dietary choices can help preserve kidney function, reduce symptoms, and prevent further damage. Understanding the importance of diet in kidney health is essential for anyone living with kidney disease.

Reducing the Workload on the Kidneys

The kidneys filter waste products and excess fluids from the blood, a process that can be significantly impacted by what we eat. By choosing foods that are easy on the kidneys, we can reduce their workload and prevent further damage. Key dietary strategies include:
- Controlling Protein Intake: While protein is essential for overall health, too much protein can create extra waste for the kidneys to filter. Managing protein intake helps reduce this burden.
- Limiting Sodium: High sodium intake can lead to fluid retention and increased blood pressure, both of which strain the kidneys. A low-sodium diet helps control blood pressure and reduce swelling.
- Balancing Potassium and Phosphorus: Maintaining proper levels of these minerals is crucial for preventing heart problems and bone disease, common complications of kidney disease.

Preventing Nutrient Imbalances

Kidney disease can disrupt the balance of essential nutrients in the body. A kidney-friendly diet helps prevent these imbalances by:

- Limiting High-Potassium Foods: Foods like bananas, oranges, and potatoes are high in potassium, which can be harmful in excess. Choosing lower-potassium alternatives helps maintain safe levels.
- Reducing Phosphorus Intake: High levels of phosphorus can weaken bones and cause heart problems. Avoiding foods like dairy products, nuts, and colas can help manage phosphorus levels.

Supporting Overall Health

A healthy diet supports not only kidney function but also overall well-being. Key components include:
- Heart Health: Kidney disease increases the risk of heart disease. A diet low in saturated fats and cholesterol, rich in fruits, vegetables, and whole grains, supports cardiovascular health.
- Blood Pressure Management: High blood pressure is both a cause and a complication of kidney disease. A diet low in sodium and rich in heart-healthy foods helps maintain normal blood pressure.
- Healthy Weight Maintenance: Maintaining a healthy weight reduces the strain on the kidneys and helps control blood pressure and blood sugar levels.

Benefits of a Vegetarian Diet

A vegetarian diet can be particularly beneficial for those with kidney disease. Plant-based diets offer numerous advantages, including:
- Lower Saturated Fat and Cholesterol: Reducing the intake of these harmful fats supports heart health and reduces inflammation.
- High in Antioxidants and Fiber: Fruits, vegetables, and whole grains provide essential nutrients and antioxidants that protect against chronic diseases.
- Naturally Low in Sodium and Phosphorus: Many plant-based foods are naturally low in these minerals, making it easier to manage their levels.

Practical Dietary Tips
Implementing a kidney-friendly diet involves practical, everyday choices. Some tips include:
- Reading Food Labels: Pay attention to sodium, potassium, and phosphorus content.
- Cooking at Home: Preparing meals at home allows you to control ingredients and avoid hidden sodium and additives.
- Staying Hydrated: Drinking the right amount of fluids is crucial. Too much or too little can strain the kidneys.
- Working with a Dietitian: A registered dietitian can provide personalized advice and meal plans tailored to your specific needs.

This cookbook is here to guide you on your dietary journey, offering delicious and kidney-friendly vegetarian recipes that support your health. By making thoughtful food choices, you can take control of your kidney health and improve your quality of life. Remember, every meal is an opportunity to nourish your body and protect your kidneys, bringing you closer to better health and well-being.

- Why a Vegetarian Diet?

Adopting a vegetarian diet can be incredibly beneficial for those managing kidney disease. Whether you're a long-time vegetarian or new to plant-based eating, the benefits of such a diet are profound and far-reaching. Here's why a vegetarian diet is a smart choice for supporting kidney health:

Lower in Protein, Easier on the Kidneys
One of the primary benefits of a vegetarian diet is it's typically lower protein content compared to a meat-based diet. While protein is essential for health, too much can be hard on the kidneys. By focusing on plant-based proteins such as beans, lentils, and tofu, you can reduce the amount of waste your kidneys need to filter, thus decreasing their workload and preventing further damage.

Reduced Sodium Intake

Processed meats and many packaged foods are often high in sodium, which can lead to increased blood pressure and fluid retention—both of which strain the kidneys. A vegetarian diet naturally emphasizes fresh fruits, vegetables, whole grains, and legumes, which are generally lower in sodium. This helps maintain healthy blood pressure levels and reduces swelling.

Balanced Potassium and Phosphorus Levels

Managing potassium and phosphorus intake is crucial for kidney health. While some plant-based foods are high in these minerals, a well-planned vegetarian diet can help keep levels in check. For example, choosing lower-potassium fruits like apples and berries, and low-phosphorus grains and vegetables, helps avoid imbalances that can lead to complications such as heart problems and bone disease.

Rich in Antioxidants and Fiber

Plant-based diets are abundant in antioxidants and fiber. Antioxidants help combat inflammation and protect against cellular damage, which is particularly important for kidney health. Fiber aids in digestion and helps regulate blood sugar levels, reducing the risk of diabetes—a leading cause of kidney disease. Fruits, vegetables, nuts, seeds, and whole grains are excellent sources of these vital nutrients.

Heart Health Benefits

Kidney disease often goes hand-in-hand with cardiovascular issues. A vegetarian diet is generally lower in saturated fats and cholesterol, which supports heart health. By focusing on plant-based foods, you can improve your cardiovascular health, reducing the risk of heart disease—a common complication of chronic kidney disease.

Weight Management

Maintaining a healthy weight is essential for kidney health. Obesity can exacerbate kidney disease and lead to other health issues such as diabetes and hypertension. A vegetarian diet, rich in whole foods and low in processed ingredients, can help you achieve and maintain a healthy weight, thus reducing the strain on your kidneys.

Sustainability and Ethical Considerations

Beyond personal health, many people choose a vegetarian diet for its environmental and ethical benefits. Plant-based diets have a lower environmental impact, using fewer natural resources and producing less pollution. Additionally, many individuals find ethical satisfaction in reducing or eliminating animal products from their diet, aligning their eating habits with their values.

Practical Tips for Adopting a Vegetarian Diet

Transitioning to a vegetarian diet, especially if it's new to you, can be smooth and enjoyable with a few practical tips:
- Start Slowly: If you're new to vegetarianism, start by incorporating more plant-based meals into your diet gradually.
- Experiment with New Recipes: Explore a variety of vegetarian dishes to keep your meals interesting and satisfying.
- Focus on Whole Foods: Emphasize whole grains, fruits, vegetables, nuts, and seeds to maximize nutritional benefits.
- Consult a Dietitian: A registered dietitian can provide personalized advice and help you create a balanced, kidney-friendly vegetarian diet.

This cookbook is designed to make your journey easier, offering delicious, nutritious, and kidney-friendly vegetarian recipes. Whether you are seeking to improve your kidney health or maintain your current lifestyle, the recipes within these pages will help you embrace the benefits of plant-based eating.

Remember, every meal is an opportunity to nourish your body and support your kidneys. By choosing a vegetarian diet, you're taking a proactive step towards better health and well-being. Enjoy the journey to a healthier, happier you with the delicious, wholesome meals in this cookbook.

- Benefits of a Plant-Based Diet for Kidney Disease

A plant-based diet offers numerous benefits for individuals managing kidney disease. By focusing on fruits, vegetables, whole grains, legumes, nuts, and seeds, you can support kidney function and overall health in several impactful ways. Here are some key benefits:

Lower Protein Load

One of the primary benefits of a plant-based diet is its generally lower protein content compared to a diet heavy in animal products. High protein intake increases the workload on the kidneys as they must filter out more waste products. Plant-based diets typically feature more moderate protein levels, primarily from sources like beans, lentils, and tofu, which are easier for the kidneys to handle.

Reduced Sodium Intake

High sodium intake is linked to high blood pressure, fluid retention, and increased strain on the kidneys. Plant-based diets naturally emphasize fresh fruits, vegetables, and whole grains, which are generally low in sodium. By avoiding processed and packaged foods often high in salt, a plant-based diet helps maintain healthy blood pressure levels and reduces the risk of fluid retention.

Balanced Potassium and Phosphorus Levels

Managing potassium and phosphorus intake is crucial for kidney health. While some plant-based foods are high in these minerals, a carefully planned plant-based diet helps keep levels in check. For example, choosing lower-potassium fruits like apples and berries and opting for low-phosphorus grains and vegetables can help avoid imbalances that may lead to complications such as heart problems and bone disease.

Rich in Antioxidants

Plant-based diets are packed with antioxidants found in fruits, vegetables, nuts, and seeds. Antioxidants help combat inflammation and protect against cellular damage, which is particularly important for kidney health.

By reducing oxidative stress, these nutrients help preserve kidney function and slow the progression of kidney disease.

High in Fiber

Fiber is abundant in plant-based foods and offers numerous benefits for kidney health. Fiber aids digestion, helps regulate blood sugar levels, and can lower cholesterol. This is particularly important for individuals with diabetes—a leading cause of kidney disease. High-fiber foods like whole grains, fruits, and vegetables also promote a feeling of fullness, aiding in weight management.

Heart Health Benefits

Kidney disease often increases the risk of cardiovascular issues. Plant-based diets are typically lower in saturated fats and cholesterol, which supports heart health. By focusing on heart-healthy foods, you can reduce the risk of heart disease—a common complication of chronic kidney disease. Additionally, the anti-inflammatory properties of many plant foods further protect cardiovascular health.

Healthy Weight Management

Maintaining a healthy weight is essential for kidney health. Obesity can exacerbate kidney disease and lead to other health issues such as diabetes and hypertension. Plant-based diets, rich in whole foods and low in processed ingredients, can help achieve and maintain a healthy weight, thus reducing the strain on your kidneys.

Improved Blood Pressure and Cholesterol Levels

A plant-based diet can help improve blood pressure and cholesterol levels, both of which are critical for kidney health. The high content of fruits, vegetables, and whole grains in a plant-based diet provides essential nutrients like potassium and magnesium, which help regulate blood pressure. Additionally, the absence of high-cholesterol animal products can lead to healthier cholesterol levels.

Enhanced Nutrient Intake
Plant-based diets offer a wide range of vitamins, minerals, and phytonutrients that support overall health and kidney function. For example, the high levels of vitamin C in many fruits and vegetables boost immune function, while magnesium and potassium help maintain normal blood pressure and heart rhythm.

Environmental and Ethical Benefits
Beyond personal health, many people choose a plant-based diet for its environmental and ethical benefits. Plant-based diets have a lower environmental impact, using fewer natural resources and producing less pollution. Additionally, reducing or eliminating animal products from your diet can align your eating habits with your ethical values, contributing to animal welfare and sustainability.

This cookbook is designed to help you embrace the benefits of a plant-based diet with delicious, kidney-friendly recipes. By making thoughtful food choices, you can support your kidney health, improve your overall well-being, and enjoy a vibrant, fulfilling diet.

Remember, every meal is an opportunity to nourish your body and protect your kidneys. With the recipes in this cookbook, you can take a proactive step towards better health and well-being, one delicious plant-based meal at a time.

Chapter 1: Kidney-Friendly Vegetarian Basics

- Key Nutrients for Kidney Health Key Nutrients for Kidney Health

Managing kidney disease through diet involves focusing on key nutrients that support kidney function and overall health. Understanding these nutrients and how to incorporate them into your diet can help you make better food choices. Here are the essential nutrients for kidney health:

Protein
Importance:
- Necessary for tissue repair and muscle maintenance.
- Produces waste products that the kidneys must filter out.

Management:
- Moderate protein intake to reduce kidney workload.
- Choose high-quality protein sources like beans, lentils, tofu, and quinoa.

Potassium
Importance:
- Regulates fluid balance, muscle contractions, and nerve signals.
- High levels can be harmful if kidneys can't filter it out properly.

Management:
- Monitor and manage intake based on your doctor's advice.
- Opt for lower-potassium fruits and vegetables like apples, berries, carrots, and green beans.

Phosphorus
Importance:
- Essential for bone health and energy production.
- Excess phosphorus can weaken bones and cause heart problems if not properly filtered by the kidneys.

Management:
- Limit high-phosphorus foods like dairy products, nuts, seeds, and certain whole grains.
- Choose lower-phosphorus options like white bread, pasta, rice, and fresh fruits and vegetables.

Sodium
Importance:
- Maintains fluid balance and blood pressure.
- Excess sodium can lead to high blood pressure and fluid retention, straining the kidneys.

Management:
   Reduce sodium intake by avoiding processed and packaged foods.
- Use herbs and spices for flavor instead of salt.

Calcium
Importance:
- Crucial for bone health.
- Kidney disease can disrupt calcium balance, leading to bone problems.

Management:
- Balance calcium intake with phosphorus management.
- Include calcium-rich but low-phosphorus foods like fortified plant milks, broccoli, and kale.

Omega-3 Fatty Acids
Importance:
- Reduce inflammation and support heart health.
- Beneficial for overall kidney health.

Sources:
- Flaxseeds, chia seeds, walnuts, and hemp seeds.

Fiber

Importance:
- Aids digestion, regulates blood sugar, and helps control cholesterol levels.
- Supports overall health and weight management.

Sources:
- Whole grains, fruits, vegetables, legumes, nuts, and seeds.

Magnesium

Importance:
- Supports muscle and nerve function, blood sugar control, and blood pressure regulation.
- Often needs careful management in kidney disease.

Sources:
- Leafy greens, whole grains, nuts, and seeds in moderation.

Iron

Importance:
- Essential for producing red blood cells and preventing anemia.
- Kidney disease can lead to iron deficiency.

Sources:
- Legumes, tofu, spinach, and iron-fortified cereals.

Vitamins

Importance:
- Various vitamins support different aspects of health, from immune function to energy production.

Management:
- B vitamins: important for energy and red blood cell production; found in whole grains, legumes, and nuts.

- Vitamin C: boosts immunity and supports tissue repair; found in fruits and vegetables.
- Vitamin D: crucial for calcium absorption and bone health; may require supplementation based on doctor's advice.

Hydration
Importance:
- Essential for overall health and kidney function.
- Proper hydration helps kidneys flush out toxins but must be balanced to avoid overloading the kidneys.

Management:
- Follow your healthcare provider's advice on fluid intake.
- Drink water and avoid sugary drinks and excessive caffeine.

This cookbook will guide you in incorporating these key nutrients into your diet through delicious, kidney-friendly vegetarian recipes. By focusing on these nutrients, you can support your kidney health and improve your overall well-being. Remember, balanced nutrition is a powerful tool in managing kidney disease and enhancing your quality of life.

- Foods to Include Foods to Include for Kidney Health

Incorporating a variety of kidney-friendly foods into your diet can help manage kidney disease and support overall health. Here are some key foods to include:

Fruits

1. Apples
   - Low in potassium and phosphorus
   - High in fiber and vitamin C

2. Berries
   - Blueberries, strawberries, and raspberries are low in potassium and rich in antioxidants

3. Grapes
   - Low in potassium and phosphorus
   - High in vitamins C and K

4. Pineapple
   - Low in potassium
   - Good source of fiber and vitamins C and B6

5. Plums
   - Low in potassium and phosphorus
   - High in vitamins C and K

Vegetables

1. Bell Peppers
   - Low in potassium and rich in vitamins A, C, and B6

2. Cabbage
   - Low in potassium and phosphorus
   - High in vitamins K and C

3. Cauliflower
   - Low in potassium
   - Good source of vitamins C and K, and fiber

4. Cucumber
   - Low in potassium and phosphorus
   - High in water content, helping with hydration

5. Lettuce
   - Low in potassium and phosphorus
   - High in vitamins A, K, and folate

6. Onions
   - Low in potassium and phosphorus

- High in antioxidants and flavonoids

7. Radishes
   - Low in potassium and phosphorus
   - High in vitamin C and fiber

8. Zucchini
   - Low in potassium and phosphorus
   - Good source of vitamins A and C

Grains and Starches

1. White Rice
   - Low in potassium and phosphorus
   - Versatile and easy to digest

2. Pasta
   - Low in potassium and phosphorus (avoid whole grain if phosphorus needs to be limited)

3. Quinoa
   - Moderate in phosphorus
   - Complete protein source and high in fiber

4. Couscous
   - Low in potassium and phosphorus
   - High in selenium and easy to prepare

5. Corn and Corn Products
   - Low in potassium and phosphorus
   - High in fiber and vitamins B and C

Legumes and Beans

1. Green Beans

- Low in potassium and phosphorus
   - Good source of vitamins A, C, and K

2. Chickpeas (in moderation)
   - Moderate in potassium and phosphorus
   - High in protein and fiber

3. Lentils (in moderation)
   - Moderate in potassium and phosphorus
   - High in protein and fiber

4. Black Beans (in moderation)
   - Moderate in potassium and phosphorus
   - High in protein and fiber

Nuts and Seeds

1. Flaxseeds
   - High in omega-3 fatty acids
   - Good source of fiber

2. Chia Seeds
   - High in omega-3 fatty acids and antioxidants
   - Good source of fiber and protein

3. Pumpkin Seeds (in moderation)
   - Moderate in potassium and phosphorus
   - High in magnesium and antioxidants

4. Walnuts
   - High in omega-3 fatty acids
   - Good source of protein and antioxidants

Dairy and Dairy Alternatives

1. Almond Milk (fortified)
   - Low in potassium and phosphorus (choose unsweetened varieties)
   - Good source of calcium and vitamin D

2. Rice Milk (fortified)
   - Low in potassium and phosphorus (choose unsweetened varieties)
   - Good source of calcium and vitamin D

Healthy Fats

1. Olive Oil
   - Heart-healthy monounsaturated fat
   - Anti-inflammatory properties

2. Avocado Oil
   - Heart-healthy monounsaturated fat
   - High smoke point for cooking

3. Coconut Oil (in moderation)
   - Contains medium-chain triglycerides (MCTs)
   - Good for cooking and baking

Herbs and Spices

1. Basil
   - Low in potassium
   - High in antioxidants

2. Parsley
   - Low in potassium and phosphorus
   - Rich in vitamins A, C, and K

3. Cilantro

- Low in potassium and phosphorus
   - High in antioxidants and vitamins A and K

4. Garlic
   - Low in potassium and phosphorus
   - Anti-inflammatory and heart-healthy properties

5. Ginger
   - Low in potassium and phosphorus
   - Anti-inflammatory and aids digestion

By incorporating these kidney-friendly foods into your diet, you can help manage kidney disease and support your overall health. The recipes in this cookbook will provide you with delicious and nutritious ways to enjoy these foods, making it easier to maintain a kidney-friendly diet.

- Foods to Avoid Foods to Avoid for Kidney Health

Managing kidney disease involves avoiding certain foods that can put additional strain on your kidneys or exacerbate your condition. Here are key foods to avoid or limit:

High-Sodium Foods

Why:
- Excess sodium increases blood pressure and fluid retention, straining the kidneys.

Examples:
- Processed and Packaged Foods: Canned soups, instant noodles, and frozen dinners
- Salty Snacks: Potato chips, pretzels, and salted nuts
- Processed Meats: Ham, bacon, sausage, and deli meats
- Condiments: Soy sauce, ketchup, pickles, and salad dressings
- Restaurant and Fast Food: Often high in sodium

High-Potassium Foods

Why:
- High potassium levels can be dangerous if kidneys cannot filter it properly.

Examples:
- Fruits: Bananas, oranges, avocados, and dried fruits
- Vegetables: Potatoes, tomatoes, spinach, and squash
- Dairy Products: Milk, yogurt, and cheese (in excess)
- Legumes: Beans, lentils, and peas (in excess)
- Nuts and Seeds: Almonds, peanuts, and sunflower seeds

High-Phosphorus Foods

Why:
- Excess phosphorus can weaken bones and cause heart problems.

Examples:
- Dairy Products: Cheese, milk, and yogurt
- Processed Foods: Colas, beer, and bottled iced tea
- Whole Grains: Brown rice, oatmeal, and whole wheat bread
- Nuts and Seeds: Almonds, walnuts, and pumpkin seeds
- Protein-Rich Foods: Organ meats, fish, and meat (in excess)

High-Protein Foods (in excess)

Why:
- High protein intake increases waste products, straining the kidneys.

Examples:
- Animal Proteins: Beef, pork, chicken, and fish (in large amounts)
- Dairy Products: Cheese, milk, and yogurt (in excess)
- Protein Supplements: Protein shakes and bars

Foods with Added Sugars

Why:
- Added sugars can lead to obesity, diabetes, and high blood pressure, all of which strain the kidneys.

Examples:
- Sugary Drinks: Sodas, sweetened coffee, and energy drinks
- Sweets: Candy, cookies, and cakes
- Processed Foods: Breakfast cereals, flavored yogurt, and snack bars

Foods High in Saturated and Trans Fats

Why:
- These fats can increase cholesterol levels and heart disease risk, which are problematic for kidney health.

Examples:
- Fried Foods: French fries, fried chicken, and doughnuts
- Baked Goods: Pastries, cookies, and pies made with hydrogenated oils
- Processed Snacks: Crackers, microwave popcorn, and chips
- High-Fat Dairy: Butter, cream, and full-fat cheese
- Red Meat: Beef, lamb, and pork (in large amounts)

Dark-Colored Sodas

Why:
- These sodas often contain high levels of phosphorus.

Examples:
- Colas: Coca-Cola, Pepsi, and root beer
- Dark Soft Drinks: Dr. Pepper, and some flavored sparkling waters

High-Oxalate Foods (for certain kidney conditions)

Why:
- High oxalate intake can lead to kidney stones in susceptible individuals.

Examples:
- Leafy Greens: Spinach, beet greens, and Swiss chard
- Nuts and Seeds: Almonds, peanuts, and sesame seeds
- Fruits: Rhubarb, figs, and star fruit
- Vegetables: Beets and sweet potatoes
- Cocoa Products: Chocolate and cocoa powder

Alcohol

Why:
- Alcohol can dehydrate the body and strain the kidneys, exacerbating kidney disease.

Examples:
- Beer
- Wine
- Spirits: Vodka, whiskey, and gin

By avoiding or limiting these foods, you can help manage your kidney disease more effectively and support your overall health. The recipes in this cookbook will provide delicious alternatives that are kind to your kidneys, making it easier to maintain a healthy, balanced diet.

- Meal Planning Tips Meal Planning Tips for Kidney Health

Effective meal planning is crucial for managing kidney disease and maintaining overall health. Here are some practical tips to help you plan kidney-friendly meals:

Understand Your Nutritional Needs
1. Consult with a Dietitian:
   - Work with a healthcare professional to understand your specific dietary needs, including protein, sodium, potassium, and phosphorus levels.

- Customize your meal plans based on your individual health conditions and preferences.

2. Read Nutrition Labels:
   - Pay close attention to sodium, potassium, and phosphorus content.
   - Look for hidden sources of these minerals in packaged and processed foods.

Focus on Fresh, Whole Foods

1. Emphasize Fruits and Vegetables:
   - Choose a variety of low-potassium and low-phosphorus options like apples, berries, bell peppers, cabbage, and lettuce.
   - Incorporate fresh produce in every meal for balanced nutrition and natural flavors.

2. Opt for Whole Grains and Low-Phosphorus Options:
   - Choose white rice, pasta, and couscous over whole grains like brown rice and whole wheat bread.
   - Explore grain alternatives like quinoa in moderation for added variety.

3. Limit Processed Foods:
   - Avoid packaged and processed foods high in sodium, phosphorus, and artificial additives.
   - Prepare meals from scratch using fresh ingredients whenever possible.

Manage Protein Intake

1. Choose Plant-Based Proteins:
   - Incorporate beans, lentils, tofu, and quinoa as protein sources.
   - Balance protein intake to avoid overburdening the kidneys.

2. Moderate Animal Proteins:
   - If you consume animal products, opt for lean cuts and smaller portions.

- Limit red meat and processed meats, which are higher in saturated fats and phosphorus.

Balance Potassium and Phosphorus

1. Monitor High-Potassium Foods:
   - Be mindful of portion sizes for high-potassium fruits and vegetables.
   - Choose lower-potassium alternatives like apples, berries, green beans, and cucumbers.

2. Limit High-Phosphorus Foods:
   - Avoid dairy products, nuts, seeds, and whole grains high in phosphorus.
   - Opt for fortified plant-based milks and low-phosphorus grains.

Control Sodium Intake

1. Cook with Fresh Ingredients:
   - Use fresh herbs, spices, and lemon juice for flavor instead of salt.
   - Avoid canned, pre-packaged, and restaurant foods high in sodium.

2. Choose Low-Sodium Alternatives:
   - Select low-sodium versions of common foods like broth, sauces, and snacks.
   - Rinse canned vegetables and beans to reduce sodium content.

Plan Balanced Meals

1. Create a Weekly Meal Plan:
   - Plan your meals in advance to ensure a balanced intake of nutrients.
   - Include a variety of fruits, vegetables, grains, and proteins in each meal.

2. Prepare Meals in Advance:
   - Batch cook and freeze meals for convenience and portion control.
   - Prepare snacks like cut fruits and vegetables to have on hand.

3. Incorporate Hydration:
   - Drink plenty of water throughout the day, following your healthcare provider's advice on fluid intake.
   - Avoid sugary drinks and excessive caffeine.

Stay Organized

1. Make a Shopping List:
   - Plan your grocery list based on your weekly meal plan.
   - Stick to the list to avoid impulse purchases and ensure you have all necessary ingredients.

2. Use Meal Prep Containers:
   - Invest in portion-controlled containers for meal prep.
   - Label containers with dates and contents to stay organized.

Enjoy Your Meals

1. Experiment with Recipes:
   - Try new kidney-friendly recipes to keep meals interesting and enjoyable.
   - Use this cookbook for delicious and nutritious meal ideas.

2. Share Meals with Loved Ones:
   - Enjoy meals with family and friends for social support and motivation.
   - Involve loved ones in meal planning and preparation for a collaborative approach.

By following these meal planning tips, you can effectively manage your kidney health while enjoying delicious, balanced meals. The recipes in this cookbook will provide you with a variety of options to make meal planning easier and more enjoyable.

Chapter 2: Breakfast Recipes

1. Apple Cinnamon Oatmeal

Ingredients:
- 1 cup rolled oats
- 2 cups water
- 1 apple, peeled and diced
- 1 teaspoon ground cinnamon
- 1 tablespoon maple syrup
- 1/4 cup unsweetened almond milk (optional)

Instructions:
1. In a medium saucepan, bring water to a boil.
2. Add oats, diced apple, and ground cinnamon.
3. Reduce heat and simmer for 10-15 minutes, stirring occasionally, until the oats are tender.
4. Stir in maple syrup and almond milk, if using.
5. Serve warm.

2. Blueberry Banana Smoothie

Ingredients:
- 1 banana
- 1/2 cup blueberries (fresh or frozen)
- 1 cup unsweetened almond milk
- 1 tablespoon chia seeds
- 1 teaspoon honey (optional)

Instructions:
1. Combine all ingredients in a blender.
2. Blend until smooth.
3. Pour into a glass and serve immediately.

3. Avocado Toast

Ingredients:
- 1 ripe avocado
- 2 slices whole grain bread (low phosphorus)
- 1/4 teaspoon black pepper
- 1/4 teaspoon red pepper flakes (optional)
- 1 tablespoon lemon juice

Instructions:
1. Toast the bread slices.
2. In a small bowl, mash the avocado with lemon juice, black pepper, and red pepper flakes.
3. Spread the avocado mixture onto the toasted bread.
4. Serve immediately.

4. Tofu Scramble

Ingredients:
- 1 block firm tofu, drained and crumbled
- 1/2 bell pepper, diced
- 1/4 onion, diced
- 1/2 teaspoon turmeric
- 1/4 teaspoon black pepper
- 1 tablespoon olive oil
- 1/4 teaspoon garlic powder

Instructions:
1. Heat olive oil in a pan over medium heat.
2. Add diced bell pepper and onion, sauté until tender.
3. Add crumbled tofu, turmeric, black pepper, and garlic powder.
4. Cook for 5-7 minutes, stirring frequently, until tofu is heated through.
5. Serve warm.

5. Berry Quinoa Breakfast Bowl

Ingredients:
- 1 cup cooked quinoa
- 1/2 cup mixed berries (blueberries, raspberries, strawberries)
- 1 tablespoon flaxseeds
- 1 tablespoon maple syrup
- 1/2 cup unsweetened almond milk

Instructions:
1. In a bowl, combine cooked quinoa, mixed berries, and flaxseeds.
2. Drizzle with maple syrup.
3. Pour almond milk over the mixture.
4. Serve immediately.

6. Green Smoothie

Ingredients:
- 1 cup spinach leaves
- 1 banana
- 1/2 cucumber, chopped
- 1 cup unsweetened almond milk
- 1 tablespoon chia seeds
- 1 teaspoon honey (optional)

Instructions:
1. Combine all ingredients in a blender.
2. Blend until smooth.
3. Pour into a glass and serve immediately.

7. Whole Grain Pancakes

Ingredients:
- 1 cup whole grain flour (low phosphorus)
- 1 tablespoon flaxseed meal
- 2 tablespoons water
- 1 cup unsweetened almond milk

- 1 tablespoon maple syrup
- 1 teaspoon baking powder
- 1/2 teaspoon vanilla extract

Instructions:
1. In a small bowl, mix flaxseed meal and water. Let sit for 5 minutes.
2. In a larger bowl, combine flour and baking powder.
3. Add almond milk, maple syrup, and vanilla extract to the flour mixture, and then add the flaxseed mixture.
4. Stir until smooth.
5. Heat a non-stick pan over medium heat.
6. Pour batter onto the pan, cooking pancakes until bubbles form and edges are set, then flip and cook until golden brown.
7. Serve warm with additional maple syrup if desired.

8. Sweet Potato Breakfast Hash

Ingredients:
- 1 large sweet potato, peeled and diced
- 1/2 bell pepper, diced
- 1/4 onion, diced
- 1 tablespoon olive oil
- 1/4 teaspoon black pepper
- 1/4 teaspoon paprika

Instructions:
1. Heat olive oil in a large skillet over medium heat.
2. Add diced sweet potato, bell pepper, and onion.
3. Season with black pepper and paprika.
4. Cook, stirring occasionally, until sweet potatoes are tender and browned, about 15-20 minutes.
5. Serve warm.

9. Chia Seed Pudding

Ingredients:
- 1/4 cup chia seeds
- 1 cup unsweetened almond milk
- 1 tablespoon maple syrup
- 1/2 teaspoon vanilla extract
- Fresh berries for topping

Instructions:
1. In a bowl, combine chia seeds, almond milk, maple syrup, and vanilla extract.
2. Stir well to combine.
3. Refrigerate for at least 2 hours or overnight, until it thickens to a pudding-like consistency.
4. Top with fresh berries before serving.

10. Almond Butter Banana Toast

Ingredients:
- 2 slices whole grain bread (low phosphorus)
- 2 tablespoons almond butter
- 1 banana, sliced
- 1/4 teaspoon cinnamon

Instructions:
1. Toast the bread slices.
2. Spread almond butter evenly on each slice.
3. Top with banana slices and sprinkle with cinnamon.
4. Serve immediately.

11. Spinach and Mushroom Breakfast Burrito

Ingredients:
- 1 whole grain tortilla (low phosphorus)
- 1 cup spinach leaves
- 1/2 cup mushrooms, sliced

- 1/4 onion, diced
- 1/4 teaspoon black pepper
- 1 tablespoon olive oil

Instructions:
1. Heat olive oil in a pan over medium heat.
2. Add onions and mushrooms, sauté until tender.
3. Add spinach and black pepper, cook until spinach is wilted.
4. Fill the tortilla with the vegetable mixture.
5. Roll up the tortilla and serve warm.

12. Mango Coconut Smoothie

Ingredients:
- 1 cup mango chunks (fresh or frozen)
- 1/2 cup unsweetened coconut milk
- 1/2 cup unsweetened almond milk
- 1 tablespoon chia seeds
- 1 teaspoon honey (optional)

Instructions:
1. Combine all ingredients in a blender.
2. Blend until smooth.
3. Pour into a glass and serve immediately.

13. Veggie Breakfast Wrap

Ingredients:
- 1 whole grain wrap (low phosphorus)
- 1/2 avocado, mashed
- 1/2 bell pepper, sliced
- 1/4 cup shredded carrots
- 1/4 cup cucumber, sliced
- 1 tablespoon lemon juice

Instructions:
1. Spread mashed avocado on the wrap.
2. Top with bell pepper, shredded carrots, and cucumber.
3. Drizzle with lemon juice.
4. Roll up the wrap and serve.

14. Oatmeal with Berries and Flax Seeds

Ingredients:
- 1 cup rolled oats
- 2 cups water
- 1/2 cup mixed berries (fresh or frozen)
- 1 tablespoon ground flaxseeds
- 1 tablespoon maple syrup

Instructions:
1. In a medium saucepan, bring water to a boil.
2. Add oats and cook, stirring occasionally, for 10-15 minutes until tender.
3. Stir in mixed berries, ground flaxseeds, and maple syrup.
4. Serve warm.

15. Pumpkin Spice Smoothie

Ingredients:
- 1/2 cup pumpkin puree
- 1 banana
- 1 cup unsweetened almond milk
- 1 tablespoon chia seeds
- 1 teaspoon pumpkin pie spice
- 1 teaspoon honey (optional)

Instructions:
1. Combine all ingredients in a blender.
2. Blend until smooth.
3. Pour into a glass and serve immediately.

16. Breakfast Quinoa with Almonds and Raisins

Ingredients:
- 1 cup cooked quinoa
- 1/4 cup sliced almonds
- 1/4 cup raisins
- 1/2 teaspoon cinnamon
- 1 tablespoon maple syrup
- 1/2 cup unsweetened almond milk

Instructions:
1. In a bowl, combine cooked quinoa, sliced almonds, raisins, and cinnamon.
2. Drizzle with maple syrup.
3. Pour almond milk over the mixture.
4. Serve immediately.

17. Tropical Smoothie Bowl

Ingredients:
- 1/2 cup pineapple chunks (fresh or frozen)
- 1/2 cup mango chunks (fresh or frozen)
- 1 banana
- 1 cup unsweetened almond milk
- 1 tablespoon chia seeds
- 1/4 cup granola (low sodium, low phosphorus)

Instructions:
1. Combine pineapple, mango, banana, and almond milk in a blender.
2. Blend until smooth.
3. Pour into a bowl and top with chia seeds and granola.
4. Serve immediately.

18. Strawberry Banana Oatmeal

Ingredients:
- 1 cup rolled oats
- 2 cups water
- 1/2 cup strawberries, sliced
- 1 banana, sliced
- 1 tablespoon maple syrup
- 1/4 cup unsweetened almond milk (optional)

Instructions:
1. In a Strawberry Banana Oatmeal (continued)

Instructions:
1. In a medium saucepan, bring water to a boil.
2. Add oats and cook, stirring occasionally, for 10-15 minutes until tender
3. Stir in sliced strawberries, banana, and maple syrup.
4. Add almond milk if desired for creaminess.
5. Serve warm.

19. Peach Chia Pudding

Ingredients:
- 1/4 cup chia seeds
- 1 cup unsweetened almond milk
- 1 tablespoon maple syrup
- 1/2 teaspoon vanilla extract
- 1 peach, diced

Instructions:
1. In a bowl, combine chia seeds, almond milk, maple syrup, and vanilla extract.
2. Stir well to combine.
3. Refrigerate for at least 2 hours or overnight, until it thickens to a pudding-like consistency.
4. Top with diced peach before serving.

20. Sweet Potato Breakfast Bowl

Ingredients:
- 1 large sweet potato, peeled and diced
- 1/4 cup walnuts, chopped
- 1 tablespoon maple syrup
- 1/4 teaspoon cinnamon
- 1/4 cup unsweetened almond milk

Instructions:
1. In a medium saucepan, bring water to a boil.
2. Add diced sweet potato and cook until tender, about 10-15 minutes.
3. Drain and mash the sweet potato.
4. Stir in walnuts, maple syrup, and cinnamon.
5. Pour almond milk over the mixture.
6. Serve warm.

Chapter 3: Lunch Recipes

1. Quinoa and Veggie Stir-Fry

Ingredients:
- 1 cup cooked quinoa
- 1/2 cup broccoli florets
- 1/2 cup bell pepper, sliced
- 1/4 cup carrots, julienned
- 1/4 cup snap peas
- 1 tablespoon olive oil
- 1 tablespoon low-sodium soy sauce
- 1 teaspoon garlic powder

Instructions:
1. Heat olive oil in a large pan over medium heat.
2. Add broccoli, bell pepper, carrots, and snap peas.
3. Stir-fry until vegetables are tender-crisp.
4. Add cooked quinoa, soy sauce, and garlic powder.
5. Stir well and cook for another 2-3 minutes.
6. Serve warm.

2. Chickpea Salad Wrap

Ingredients:
- 1 can chickpeas, drained and rinsed
- 1/4 cup celery, diced
- 1/4 cup red onion, diced
- 2 tablespoons vegan mayonnaise
- 1 teaspoon lemon juice
- 1/4 teaspoon black pepper
- 2 whole grain wraps (low phosphorus)
- Lettuce leaves

Instructions:

1. In a bowl, mash chickpeas until chunky.
2. Add celery, red onion, vegan mayonnaise, lemon juice, and black pepper.
3. Mix well.
4. Place lettuce leaves on wraps and top with chickpea mixture.
5. Roll up the wraps and serve.

3. Lentil and Vegetable Soup

Ingredients:
- 1 cup dried lentils, rinsed
- 1 carrot, diced
- 1 celery stalk, diced
- 1/2 onion, diced
- 2 garlic cloves, minced
- 1 can diced tomatoes, no salt added
- 4 cups low-sodium vegetable broth
- 1 tablespoon olive oil
- 1 teaspoon thyme
- 1/2 teaspoon black pepper

Instructions:
1. Heat olive oil in a large pot over medium heat.
2. Add onion, garlic, carrot, and celery. Sauté until vegetables are tender.
3. Add lentils, diced tomatoes, vegetable broth, thyme, and black pepper.
4. Bring to a boil, then reduce heat and simmer for 30-40 minutes until lentils are tender.
5. Serve warm.

4. Spinach and Avocado Salad

Ingredients:
- 2 cups spinach leaves
- 1 avocado, diced
- 1/4 cup cherry tomatoes, halved
- 1/4 cup cucumber, sliced

- 1 tablespoon lemon juice
- 1 tablespoon olive oil
- 1/4 teaspoon black pepper

Instructions:
1. In a large bowl, combine spinach, avocado, cherry tomatoes, and cucumber.
2. In a small bowl, whisk together lemon juice, olive oil, and black pepper.
3. Drizzle dressing over salad and toss to coat.
4. Serve immediately.

5. Veggie Burger

Ingredients:
- 1 can black beans, drained and rinsed
- 1/4 cup breadcrumbs (low sodium)
- 1/4 cup red onion, diced
- 1 garlic clove, minced
- 1 teaspoon cumin
- 1/2 teaspoon black pepper
- 1 tablespoon olive oil
- 2 whole grain buns (low phosphorus)
- Lettuce, tomato, and avocado slices for topping

Instructions:
1. In a bowl, mash black beans until chunky.
2. Add breadcrumbs, red onion, garlic, cumin, and black pepper. Mix well.
3. Form mixture into patties.
4. Heat olive oil in a pan over medium heat.
5. Cook patties for 4-5 minutes on each side, until golden brown.
6. Serve on buns with lettuce, tomato, and avocado slices.

6. Stuffed Bell Peppers

Ingredients:

- 4 bell peppers, tops cut off and seeds removed
- 1 cup cooked quinoa
- 1/2 cup black beans, drained and rinsed
- 1/2 cup corn kernels
- 1/4 cup red onion, diced
- 1 tablespoon olive oil
- 1 teaspoon cumin
- 1/2 teaspoon paprika
- 1/4 teaspoon black pepper

Instructions:
1. Preheat the oven to 375°F (190°C).
2. In a bowl, combine cooked quinoa, black beans, corn, red onion, olive oil, cumin, paprika, and black pepper.
3. Stuff bell peppers with the quinoa mixture.
4. Place stuffed peppers in a baking dish and cover with foil.
5. Bake for 30-35 minutes, until peppers are tender.
6. Serve warm.

7. Zucchini Noodles with Pesto

Ingredients:
- 2 large zucchinis, spiralized into noodles
- 1/2 cup fresh basil leaves
- 1/4 cup pine nuts
- 1 garlic clove
- 1/4 cup olive oil
- 1 tablespoon lemon juice
- 1/4 teaspoon black pepper

Instructions:
1. In a food processor, combine basil, pine nuts, garlic, olive oil, lemon juice, and black pepper. Blend until smooth to make the pesto.
2. In a large pan, lightly sauté zucchini noodles over medium heat for 2-3 minutes.

3. Remove from heat and toss with pesto.
4. Serve immediately.

8. Cucumber and Hummus Sandwich

Ingredients:
- 2 slices whole grain bread (low phosphorus)
- 1/4 cup hummus
- 1/2 cucumber, sliced
- 1/4 teaspoon black pepper
- Lettuce leaves

Instructions:
1. Spread hummus evenly on each slice of bread.
2. Top with cucumber slices, black pepper, and lettuce leaves.
3. Place the other slice of bread on top.
4. Serve immediately.

9. Vegetable Stir-Fry with Brown Rice

Ingredients:
- 1 cup cooked brown rice
- 1/2 cup broccoli florets
- 1/2 cup bell pepper, sliced
- 1/4 cup carrots, julienned
- 1/4 cup snap peas
- 1 tablespoon olive oil
- 1 tablespoon low-sodium soy sauce
- 1 teaspoon ginger, grated

Instructions:
1. Heat olive oil in a large pan over medium heat.
2. Add broccoli, bell pepper, carrots, and snap peas.
3. Stir-fry until vegetables are tender-crisp.
4. Add cooked brown rice, soy sauce, and grated ginger.

5. Stir well and cook for another 2-3 minutes.
6. Serve warm.

10. Butternut Squash Soup

Ingredients:
- 1 medium butternut squash, peeled, seeded, and diced
- 1 carrot, diced
- 1/2 onion, diced
- 2 garlic cloves, minced
- 4 cups low-sodium vegetable broth
- 1 tablespoon olive oil
- 1/2 teaspoon thyme
- 1/4 teaspoon black pepper

Instructions:
1. Heat olive oil in a large pot over medium heat.
2. Add onion and garlic. Sauté until tender.
3. Add diced butternut squash and carrot. Cook for 5 minutes.
4. Add vegetable broth, thyme, and black pepper. Bring to a boil.
5. Reduce heat and simmer for 20-25 minutes, until vegetables are tender.
6. Puree the soup with an immersion blender until smooth.
7. Serve warm.

11. Mediterranean Chickpea Salad

Ingredients:
- 1 can chickpeas, drained and rinsed
- 1/2 cup cherry tomatoes, halved
- 1/2 cucumber, diced
- 1/4 cup red onion, diced
- 1/4 cup kalamata olives, pitted and sliced
- 2 tablespoons olive oil
- 1 tablespoon lemon juice
- 1/4 teaspoon black pepper

Instructions:
1. In a large bowl, combine chickpeas, cherry tomatoes, cucumber, red onion, and olives.
2. In a small bowl, whisk together olive oil, lemon juice, and black pepper.
3. Drizzle dressing over salad and toss to coat.
4. Serve immediately.

12. Roasted Veggie and Quinoa Bowl

Ingredients:
- 1 cup cooked quinoa
- 1 cup mixed vegetables (zucchini, bell pepper, carrots, and broccoli)
- 1 tablespoon olive oil
- 1/4 teaspoon black pepper
- 1/2 teaspoon garlic powder
- 1 tablespoon lemon juice

Instructions:
1. Preheat the oven to 400°F (200°C).
2. Toss mixed vegetables with olive oil, black pepper, and garlic powder.
3. Spread vegetables on a baking sheet and roast for 20-25 minutes, until tender and slightly caramelized.
4. In a bowl, combine cooked quinoa, roasted vegetables, and lemon juice.
5. Serve warm.

13. Black Bean and Corn Salad

Ingredients:
- 1 can black beans, drained and rinsed
- 1/2 cup corn kernels
- 1/4 cup red bell pepper, diced
- 1/4 cup red onion, diced
- 1/4 cup cilantro, chopped
- 1 tablespoon lime juice

- 1 tablespoon olive oil
- 1/4 teaspoon cumin
- 1/4 teaspoon black pepper

Instructions:
1. In a large bowl,1. In a large bowl, combine black beans, corn, red bell pepper, red onion, and cilantro.
2. In a small bowl, whisk together lime juice, olive oil, cumin, and black pepper.
3. Drizzle dressing over the salad and toss to coat.
4. Serve immediately.

14. Tofu and Vegetable Stir-Fry

Ingredients:
- 1 block firm tofu, drained and cubed
- 1/2 cup broccoli florets
- 1/2 cup bell pepper, sliced
- 1/4 cup carrots, julienned
- 1/4 cup snap peas
- 1 tablespoon olive oil
- 1 tablespoon low-sodium soy sauce
- 1 teaspoon ginger, grated

Instructions:
1. Heat olive oil in a large pan over medium heat.
2. Add tofu and cook until golden brown on all sides.
3. Remove tofu and set aside.
4. In the same pan, add broccoli, bell pepper, carrots, and snap peas.
5. Stir-fry until vegetables are tender-crisp.
6. Add tofu back to the pan, along with soy sauce and grated ginger.
7. Stir well and cook for another 2-3 minutes.
8. Serve warm.

15. Avocado and Tomato Sandwich

Ingredients:
- 2 slices whole grain bread (low phosphorus)
- 1 avocado, sliced
- 1 tomato, sliced
- 1/4 teaspoon black pepper
- 1 tablespoon lemon juice
- Lettuce leaves

Instructions:
1. Toast the bread slices if desired.
2. Arrange avocado and tomato slices on one slice of bread.
3. Sprinkle with black pepper and lemon juice.
4. Add lettuce leaves and top with the other slice of bread.
5. Serve immediately.

16. Sweet Potato and Black Bean Tacos

Ingredients:
- 1 large sweet potato, peeled and diced
- 1 can black beans, drained and rinsed
- 1/4 cup red onion, diced
- 1 tablespoon olive oil
- 1 teaspoon cumin
- 1/2 teaspoon paprika
- 1/4 teaspoon black pepper
- Corn tortillas
- Fresh cilantro, chopped

Instructions:
1. Preheat the oven to 400°F (200°C).
2. Toss diced sweet potato with olive oil, cumin, paprika, and black pepper.
3. Spread sweet potatoes on a baking sheet and roast for 20-25 minutes, until tender.
4. In a pan, heat black beans with red onion until warmed through.

5. Assemble tacos by filling corn tortillas with roasted sweet potato, black beans, and red onion mixture.
6. Top with fresh cilantro.
7. Serve immediately.

17. Broccoli and Chickpea Bowl

Ingredients:
- 1 cup cooked brown rice
- 1 cup broccoli florets
- 1 can chickpeas, drained and rinsed
- 1 tablespoon olive oil
- 1 tablespoon tahini
- 1 tablespoon lemon juice
- 1/4 teaspoon black pepper

Instructions:
1. Steam broccoli until tender.
2. In a bowl, combine cooked brown rice, steamed broccoli, and chickpeas.
3. In a small bowl, whisk together olive oil, tahini, lemon juice, and black pepper.
4. Drizzle dressing over the rice bowl and toss to coat.
5. Serve warm.

18. Greek Salad

Ingredients:
- 1 cup cherry tomatoes, halved
- 1 cucumber, diced
- 1/4 cup red onion, sliced
- 1/4 cup kalamata olives, pitted and sliced
- 1/4 cup feta cheese, crumbled (optional)
- 2 tablespoons olive oil
- 1 tablespoon red wine vinegar
- 1/4 teaspoon oregano

- 1/4 teaspoon black pepper

Instructions:
1. In a large bowl, combine cherry tomatoes, cucumber, red onion, and kalamata olives.
2. In a small bowl, whisk together olive oil, red wine vinegar, oregano, and black pepper.
3. Drizzle dressing over the salad and toss to coat.
4. Sprinkle with feta cheese, if using.
5. Serve immediately.

19. Mushroom and Spinach Quesadilla

Ingredients:
- 2 whole grain tortillas (low phosphorus)
- 1 cup mushrooms, sliced
- 1 cup spinach leaves
- 1/4 cup vegan cheese, shredded
- 1 tablespoon olive oil

Instructions:
1. Heat olive oil in a pan over medium heat.
2. Add mushrooms and cook until tender.
3. Add spinach and cook until wilted.
4. Remove from heat.
5. Place one tortilla in a clean pan over medium heat.
6. Spread mushroom and spinach mixture over the tortilla.
7. Sprinkle with vegan cheese and top with the second tortilla.
8. Cook until the bottom tortilla is golden brown, then flip and cook until the other side is golden brown.
9. Cut into wedges and serve warm.

20. Roasted Cauliflower and Chickpea Salad

Ingredients:

- 1 head cauliflower, cut into florets
- 1 can chickpeas, drained and rinsed
- 1 tablespoon olive oil
- 1 teaspoon cumin
- 1/4 teaspoon black pepper
- 4 cups mixed greens
- 1/4 cup tahini
- 1 tablespoon lemon juice
- 1 tablespoon water

Instructions:
1. Preheat the oven to 400°F (200°C).
2. Toss cauliflower florets and chickpeas with olive oil, cumin, and black pepper.
3. Spread on a baking sheet and roast for 20-25 minutes, until tender and golden brown.
4. In a large bowl, combine roasted cauliflower, chickpeas, and mixed greens.
5. In a small bowl, whisk together tahini, lemon juice, and water to make the dressing.
6. Drizzle dressing over the salad and toss to coat.
7. Serve immediately.

Chapter 4: Dinner Recipes

1. Eggplant and Tomato Stew

Ingredients:
- 1 large eggplant, diced
- 1 can diced tomatoes, no salt added
- 1/2 onion, diced
- 2 garlic cloves, minced
- 1 tablespoon olive oil
- 1 teaspoon cumin
- 1/2 teaspoon paprika
- 1/4 teaspoon black pepper
- 1/4 cup fresh parsley, chopped

Instructions:
1. Heat olive oil in a large pot over medium heat.
2. Add onion and garlic, sauté until tender.
3. Add diced eggplant, diced tomatoes, cumin, paprika, and black pepper.
4. Bring to a boil, then reduce heat and simmer for 20-25 minutes, until eggplant is tender.
5. Stir in fresh parsley.
6. Serve warm.

2. Lentil and Sweet Potato Curry

Ingredients:
- 1 cup dried lentils, rinsed
- 1 large sweet potato, peeled and diced
- 1 can coconut milk, light
- 1/2 onion, diced
- 2 garlic cloves, minced
- 1 tablespoon curry powder
- 1 tablespoon olive oil
- 1/4 teaspoon black pepper

- 4 cups low-sodium vegetable broth

Instructions:
1. Heat olive oil in a large pot over medium heat.
2. Add onion and garlic, sauté until tender.
3. Add curry powder and cook for 1 minute.
4. Add lentils, sweet potato, coconut milk, black pepper, and vegetable broth.
5. Bring to a boil, then reduce heat and simmer for 30-35 minutes, until lentils and sweet potato are tender.
6. Serve warm.

3. Baked Stuffed Portobello Mushrooms

Ingredients:
- 4 large portobello mushrooms, stems removed
- 1/2 cup quinoa, cooked
- 1/2 cup spinach, chopped
- 1/4 cup sun-dried tomatoes, chopped
- 2 tablespoons pine nuts
- 1 tablespoon olive oil
- 1 garlic clove, minced
- 1/4 teaspoon black pepper

Instructions:
1. Preheat the oven to 375°F (190°C).
2. In a bowl, combine cooked quinoa, spinach, sun-dried tomatoes, pine nuts, olive oil, garlic, and black pepper.
3. Stuff portobello mushrooms with the quinoa mixture.
4. Place mushrooms on a baking sheet and bake for 20-25 minutes, until tender.
5. Serve warm.

4. Vegetable Paella

Ingredients:
- 1 cup brown rice
- 1 red bell pepper, sliced
- 1 yellow bell pepper, sliced
- 1/2 cup green beans, trimmed
- 1/2 cup peas
- 1/2 onion, diced
- 2 garlic cloves, minced
- 1 can diced tomatoes, no salt added
- 4 cups low-sodium vegetable broth
- 1 tablespoon olive oil
- 1 teaspoon smoked paprika
- 1/4 teaspoon saffron threads (optional)
- 1/4 teaspoon black pepper

Instructions:
1. Heat olive oil in a large pan over medium heat.
2. Add onion and garlic, sauté until tender.
3. Add brown rice, smoked paprika, and saffron (if using), stir well.
4. Add diced tomatoes and vegetable broth, bring to a boil.
5. Reduce heat, cover, and simmer for 30-35 minutes, until rice is tender.
6. Add bell peppers, green beans, and peas, cook for another 10 minutes.
7. Serve warm.

5. Cauliflower Tacos

Ingredients:
- 1 head cauliflower, cut into florets
- 1 tablespoon olive oil
- 1 teaspoon cumin
- 1/2 teaspoon paprika
- 1/4 teaspoon black pepper
- Corn tortillas
- Fresh cilantro, chopped
- Lime wedges for serving

Instructions:
1. Preheat the oven to 400°F (200°C).
2. Toss cauliflower florets with olive oil, cumin, paprika, and black pepper.
3. Spread on a baking sheet and roast for 20-25 minutes, until tender.
4. Serve roasted cauliflower in corn tortillas, topped with fresh cilantro and lime wedges.

6. Spinach and Tofu Stir-Fry

Ingredients:
- 1 block firm tofu, drained and cubed
- 2 cups spinach leaves
- 1/2 cup bell pepper, sliced
- 1/4 cup red onion, sliced
- 2 garlic cloves, minced
- 1 tablespoon olive oil
- 1 tablespoon low-sodium soy sauce
- 1/4 teaspoon black pepper

Instructions:
1. Heat olive oil in a large pan over medium heat.
2. Add tofu and cook until golden brown on all sides.
3. Remove tofu and set aside.
4. In the same pan, add garlic and red onion, sauté until tender.
5. Add bell pepper and spinach, cook until spinach is wilted.
6. Return tofu to the pan, add soy sauce and black pepper.
7. Stir well and cook for another 2-3 minutes.
8. Serve warm.

7. Stuffed Zucchini Boats

Ingredients:
- 4 zucchinis, halved lengthwise and seeds scooped out
- 1 cup cooked quinoa

- 1/2 cup cherry tomatoes, halved
- 1/4 cup red onion, diced
- 1/4 cup black beans, drained and rinsed
- 1 tablespoon olive oil
- 1 teaspoon Italian seasoning
- 1/4 teaspoon black pepper

Instructions:
1. Preheat the oven to 375°F (190°C).
2. In a bowl, combine cooked quinoa, cherry tomatoes, red onion, black beans, olive oil, Italian seasoning, and black pepper.
3. Stuff zucchini halves with the quinoa mixture.
4. Place stuffed zucchinis in a baking dish and cover with foil.
5. Bake for 20-25 minutes, until zucchinis are tender.
6. Serve warm.

8. Vegan Shepherd's Pie

Ingredients:
- 4 large potatoes, peeled and diced
- 1/2 cup almond milk (unsweetened)
- 1 tablespoon olive oil
- 1/2 onion, diced
- 2 garlic cloves, minced
- 1 cup lentils, cooked
- 1 cup mixed vegetables (carrots, peas, corn)
- 1 tablespoon tomato paste
- 1 teaspoon thyme
- 1/4 teaspoon black pepper

Instructions:
1. Preheat the oven to 375°F (190°C).
2. Boil potatoes until tender, then mash with almond milk.
3. Heat olive oil in a pan over medium heat.
4. Add onion and garlic, sauté until tender.

5. Add cooked lentils, mixed vegetables, tomato paste, thyme, and black pepper. Stir well and cook for 5 minutes.
6. Transfer lentil mixture to a baking dish and spread mashed potatoes on top.
7. Bake for 20-25 minutes, until golden brown.
8. Serve warm.

9. Ratatouille

Ingredients:
- 1 eggplant, diced
- 1 zucchini, diced
- 1 red bell pepper, diced
- 1 yellow bell pepper, diced
- 1/2 onion, diced
- 2 garlic cloves, minced
- 1 can diced tomatoes, no salt added
- 1 tablespoon olive oil
- 1 teaspoon thyme
- 1/4 teaspoon black pepper

Instructions:
1. Heat olive oil in a large pot over medium heat.
2. Add onion and garlic, sauté until tender.
3. Add eggplant, zucchini, bell peppers, and diced tomatoes.
4. Stir in thyme and black pepper.
5. Bring to a boil, then reduce heat and simmer for 25-30 minutes, until vegetables are tender.
6. Serve warm.

10. Chickpea and Spinach Curry

Ingredients:
- 1 can chickpeas, drained and rinsed
- 2 cups spinach leaves

- 1/2 onion, diced
- 2 garlic cloves, minced
- 1 can coconut milk, light
- 1 tablespoon curry powder
- 1 tablespoon olive oil
- 1/4 teaspoon black pepper

Instructions:
1. Heat olive oil in a large pot over medium heat.
2. Add onion and garlic, sauté until tender.
3. Add curry powder and cook for 1 minute.
4. Add chickpeas, coconut milk, and black pepper.
5. Bring to a boil, then reduce heat and simmer for 10-15 minutes.
6. Stir in spinach until wilted.
7. Serve warm.

11. Spaghetti Squash with Marinara Sauce

Ingredients:
- 1 spaghetti squash, halved and seeded
- 2 cups marinara sauce (low sodium)
- 1/4 cup fresh basil, chopped
- 1/4 teaspoon black pepper

Instructions:
1. Preheat the oven to 400°F (200°C).
2. Place spaghetti squash halves cut-side down on a baking sheet.
3. Bake for 30-35 minutes, until tender.
4. Scrape the flesh with a fork to create spaghetti-like strands.
5. Heat marinara sauce in a pan over medium heat.
6. Serve spaghetti squash topped with marinara sauce and fresh basil.

12. Black Bean and Vegetable Enchiladas

Ingredients:

- 1 can black beans, drained and rinsed
- 1/2 cup corn kernels
- 1/2 bell pepper, diced
- 1/2 onion, diced
- 2 garlic cloves, minced
- 1 teaspoon cumin
- 1/2 teaspoon chili powder
- 1/4 teaspoon black pepper
- 8 whole grain tortillas (low phosphorus)
- 1 cup enchilada sauce (low sodium)
- 1/2 cup vegan cheese, shredded (optional)

Instructions:
1. Preheat the oven to 375°F (190°C).
2. In a pan, sauté bell pepper, onion, and garlic until tender.
3. Add black beans, corn, cumin, chili powder, and black pepper. Cook for 5 minutes.
4. Spread a thin layer of enchilada sauce on the bottom of a baking dish.
5. Fill each tortilla with the bean mixture, roll up, and place seam-side down in the baking dish.
6. Pour remaining enchilada sauce over the top and sprinkle with vegan cheese, if using.
7. Bake for 20-25 minutes, until heated through and the cheese is melted.
8. Serve warm.

13. Lentil and Mushroom Loaf

Ingredients:
- 1 cup brown lentils, cooked
- 1 cup mushrooms, finely chopped
- 1/2 onion, diced
- 2 garlic cloves, minced
- 1/2 cup oats
- 1/4 cup tomato paste
- 1 tablespoon soy sauce

- 1 teaspoon thyme
- 1/2 teaspoon black pepper

Instructions:
1. Preheat the oven to 375°F (190°C).
2. In a pan, sauté mushrooms, onion, and garlic until tender.
3. In a large bowl, combine cooked lentils, sautéed mushrooms mixture, oats, tomato paste, soy sauce, thyme, and black pepper.
4. Transfer mixture to a loaf pan lined with parchment paper.
5. Bake for 30-35 minutes, until firm and golden brown.
6. Serve warm.

14. Butternut Squash and Sage Risotto

Ingredients:
- 1 butternut squash, peeled and diced
- 1 cup arborio rice
- 1/2 onion, diced
- 2 garlic cloves, minced
- 4 cups low-sodium vegetable broth
- 1/4 cup nutritional yeast
- 1 tablespoon olive oil
- 1 tablespoon fresh sage, chopped
- 1/4 teaspoon black pepper

Instructions:
1. In a large pot, heat olive oil over medium heat.
2. Add onion and garlic, sauté until tender.
3. Add arborio rice and cook for 1-2 minutes.
4. Stir in diced butternut squash.
5. Add vegetable broth, 1/2 cup at a time, stirring frequently and allowing liquid to absorb before adding more.
6. Continue until rice and squash are tender and creamy.
7. Stir in nutritional yeast, sage, and black pepper.
8. Serve warm.

15. Quinoa Stuffed Bell Peppers

Ingredients:
- 4 bell peppers, halved and seeds removed
- 1 cup quinoa, cooked
- 1 can black beans, drained and rinsed
- 1/2 cup corn kernels
- 1/2 onion, diced
- 2 garlic cloves, minced
- 1 teaspoon cumin
- 1/2 teaspoon chili powder
- 1/4 teaspoon black pepper
- 1/4 cup cilantro, chopped

Instructions:
1. Preheat the oven to 375°F (190°C).
2. In a bowl, combine cooked quinoa, black beans, corn, onion, garlic, cumin, chili powder, black pepper, and cilantro.
3. Fill each bell pepper half with the quinoa mixture.
4. Place stuffed bell peppers in a baking dish.
5. Cover with foil and bake for 25-30 minutes, until peppers are tender.
6. Serve warm.

16. Sweet Potato and Black Bean Chili

Ingredients:
- 2 large sweet potatoes, peeled and diced
- 1 can black beans, drained and rinsed
- 1 can diced tomatoes, no salt added
- 1/2 onion, diced
- 2 garlic cloves, minced
- 1 tablespoon olive oil
- 1 tablespoon chili powder
- 1 teaspoon cumin
- 1/4 teaspoon black pepper

- 4 cups low-sodium vegetable broth

Instructions:
1. In a large pot, heat olive oil over medium heat.
2. Add onion and garlic, sauté until tender.
3. Add sweet potatoes, black beans, diced tomatoes, chili powder, cumin, black pepper, and vegetable broth.
4. Bring to a boil, then reduce heat and simmer for 20-25 minutes, until sweet potatoes are tender.
5. Serve warm.

17. Vegetable and Lentil Curry

Ingredients:
- 1 cup brown lentils, cooked
- 2 cups mixed vegetables (carrots, peas, bell peppers)
- 1/2 onion, diced
- 2 garlic cloves, minced
- 1 can coconut milk, light
- 1 tablespoon curry powder
- 1 tablespoon olive oil
- 1/4 teaspoon black pepper

Instructions:
1. Heat olive oil in a large pot over medium heat.
2. Add onion and garlic, sauté until tender.
3. Add mixed vegetables and cook for 5 minutes.
4. Stir in cooked lentils, coconut milk, curry powder, and black pepper.
5. Bring to a boil, then reduce heat and simmer for 15-20 minutes.
6. Serve warm.

18. Spinach and Chickpea Curry

Ingredients:
- 1 can chickpeas, drained and rinsed

- 2 cups spinach leaves
- 1/2 onion, diced
- 2 garlic cloves, minced
- 1 can diced tomatoes, no salt added
- 1 tablespoon curry powder
- 1 tablespoon olive oil
- 1/4 teaspoon black pepper

Instructions:
1. Heat olive oil in a large pot over medium heat.
2. Add onion and garlic, sauté until tender.
3. Add chickpeas, spinach, diced tomatoes, curry powder, and black pepper.
4. Cook for 10-15 minutes, until spinach is wilted.
5. Serve warm.

19. Mushroom and Spinach Lasagna

Ingredients:
- 9 whole grain lasagna noodles (low phosphorus)
- 2 cups mushrooms, sliced
- 2 cups spinach leaves
- 1/2 onion, diced
- 2 garlic cloves, minced
- 2 cups marinara sauce (low sodium)
- 1 cup vegan ricotta cheese
- 1/2 cup vegan mozzarella cheese, shredded
- 1 tablespoon olive oil
- 1/4 teaspoon black pepper

Instructions:
1. Preheat the oven to 375°F (190°C).
2. Cook lasagna noodles according to package instructions.
3. In a pan, sauté mushrooms, onion, and garlic until tender.
4. In a bowl, combine sautéed mushrooms mixture, spinach, and black pepper.

5. In a baking dish, layer marinara sauce, lasagna noodles, mushroom-spinach mixture, and vegan ricotta cheese. Repeat layers.
6. Top with vegan mozzarella cheese.
7. Cover with foil and bake for 30-35 minutes, until heated through.
8. Serve warm.

20. Tofu and Vegetable Kebabs

Ingredients:
- 1 block firm tofu, cubed
- 1 bell pepper, diced
- 1 zucchini, diced
- 1/2 onion, diced
- 1/4 cup soy sauce
- 1/4 cup maple syrup
- 1 tablespoon olive oil
- 1 teaspoon garlic powder
- 1/2 teaspoon black pepper
- Wooden skewers, soaked in water

Instructions:
1. In a bowl, combine soy sauce, maple syrup, olive oil, garlic powder, and black pepper.
2. Add tofu, bell pepper, zucchini, and onion to the bowl. Marinate for at least 30 minutes.
3. Thread marinated tofu and vegetables onto soaked wooden skewers.
4. Grill or bake kebabs until tofu is golden brown and vegetables are tender.
5. Serve warm.

Chapter 5: Snacks and Sides

1. Hummus and Veggie Sticks

Ingredients:
- 1 can chickpeas, drained and rinsed
- 2 tablespoons tahini
- 2 tablespoons lemon juice
- 1 garlic clove, minced
- 1/4 teaspoon cumin
- 1/4 teaspoon paprika
- Carrot, cucumber, and bell pepper sticks for dipping

Instructions:
1. Blend chickpeas, tahini, lemon juice, garlic, cumin, and paprika in a food processor until smooth.
2. Serve hummus with veggie sticks for dipping.

2. Roasted Chickpeas

Ingredients:
- 1 can chickpeas, drained and rinsed
- 1 tablespoon olive oil
- 1/2 teaspoon cumin
- 1/2 teaspoon paprika
- 1/4 teaspoon garlic powder
- 1/4 teaspoon salt

Instructions:
1. Preheat the oven to 400°F (200°C).
2. Pat chickpeas dry with a paper towel.
3. Toss chickpeas with olive oil, cumin, paprika, garlic powder, and salt.
4. Spread chickpeas on a baking sheet and bake for 20-25 minutes, until crispy.

3. Greek Yogurt Parfait

Ingredients:
- 1 cup Greek yogurt
- 1/2 cup mixed berries
- 2 tablespoons almonds, chopped
- 1 tablespoon honey

Instructions:
1. Layer Greek yogurt, mixed berries, and chopped almonds in a glass.
2. Drizzle with honey before serving.

4. Vegetable Soup

Ingredients:
- 4 cups low-sodium vegetable broth
- 1 can diced tomatoes, no salt added
- 1 carrot, diced
- 1 celery stalk, diced
- 1/2 onion, diced
- 1 garlic clove, minced
- 1/2 cup green beans, chopped
- 1/2 cup spinach leaves
- 1/4 teaspoon black pepper
- 1/4 teaspoon thyme

Instructions:
1. In a large pot, combine vegetable broth, diced tomatoes, carrot, celery, onion, and garlic.
2. Bring to a boil, then reduce heat and simmer for 20-25 minutes, until vegetables are tender.
3. Add green beans, spinach, black pepper, and thyme. Cook for another 5 minutes.
4. Serve warm.

5. Cucumber Salad

Ingredients:
- 2 cucumbers, thinly sliced
- 1/4 cup red onion, thinly sliced
- 2 tablespoons apple cider vinegar
- 1 tablespoon olive oil
- 1 teaspoon honey
- 1/4 teaspoon black pepper
- Fresh dill, chopped

Instructions:
1. In a bowl, combine cucumbers and red onion.
2. In a separate bowl, whisk together apple cider vinegar, olive oil, honey, black pepper, and chopped dill.
3. Pour dressing over cucumber mixture and toss to coat.
4. Refrigerate for at least 30 minutes before serving.

6. Baked Sweet Potato Fries

Ingredients:
- 2 sweet potatoes, cut into fries
- 1 tablespoon olive oil
- 1/2 teaspoon paprika
- 1/4 teaspoon garlic powder
- 1/4 teaspoon black pepper

Instructions:
1. Preheat the oven to 425°F (220°C).
2. Toss sweet potato fries with olive oil, paprika, garlic powder, and black pepper.
3. Spread fries in a single layer on a baking sheet.
4. Bake for 20-25 minutes, flipping halfway through, until crispy.

7. Brown Rice and Lentil Pilaf

Ingredients:
- 1 cup brown rice, cooked
- 1/2 cup brown lentils, cooked
- 1/4 cup almonds, chopped
- 1/4 cup dried cranberries
- 1 tablespoon olive oil
- 1/2 teaspoon cumin
- 1/4 teaspoon cinnamon
- 1/4 teaspoon black pepper

Instructions:
1. In a large pan, heat olive oil over medium heat.
2. Add cooked brown rice, brown lentils, almonds, dried cranberries, cumin, cinnamon, and black pepper.
3. Stir well and cook for 5 minutes, until heated through.
4. Serve warm.

8. Steamed Asparagus with Lemon

Ingredients:
- 1 bunch asparagus, trimmed
- 1 tablespoon olive oil
- 1 tablespoon lemon juice
- 1/4 teaspoon black pepper

Instructions:
1. Steam asparagus until tender.
2. Drizzle with olive oil and lemon juice.
3. Season with black pepper before serving.

9. Caprese Salad Skewers

Ingredients:
- Cherry tomatoes

- Fresh basil leaves
- Mozzarella balls
- Balsamic glaze

Instructions:
1. Thread cherry tomatoes, fresh basil leaves, and mozzarella balls onto skewers.
2. Drizzle with balsamic glaze before serving.

10. Apple and Almond Butter Slices

Ingredients:
- 1 apple, sliced
- 2 tablespoons almond butter
- 1 tablespoon honey
- 1 tablespoon chopped almonds

Instructions:
1. Spread almond butter on apple slices.
2. Drizzle with honey and sprinkle with chopped almonds.

11. Edamame Salad

Ingredients:
- 1 cup shelled edamame, cooked
- 1/2 cup cucumber, diced
- 1/4 cup red bell pepper, diced
- 2 tablespoons red onion, diced
- 2 tablespoons rice vinegar
- 1 tablespoon sesame oil
- 1 teaspoon soy sauce
- 1/2 teaspoon ginger, grated
- 1/4 teaspoon black pepper
- Sesame seeds for garnish

Instructions:
1. In a bowl, combine cooked edamame, cucumber, red bell pepper, and red onion.
2. In a separate bowl, whisk together rice vinegar, sesame oil, soy sauce, ginger, and black pepper.
3. Pour dressing over edamame mixture and toss to coat.
4. Sprinkle with sesame seeds before serving.

12. Stuffed Mini Bell Peppers

Ingredients:
- 12 mini bell peppers, halved and seeds removed
- 1 cup quinoa, cooked
- 1/2 cup black beans, drained and rinsed
- 1/2 cup corn kernels
- 1/4 cup red onion, diced
- 1/4 cup cilantro, chopped
- 1/2 teaspoon cumin
- 1/4 teaspoon chili powder
- 1/4 teaspoon black pepper
- 1/4 cup vegan cheese, shredded (optional)

Instructions:
1. Preheat the oven to 375°F (190°C).
2. In a bowl, combine cooked quinoa, black beans, corn, red onion, cilantro, cumin, chili powder, and black pepper.
3. Fill each mini bell pepper half with the quinoa mixture.
4. Place stuffed peppers on a baking sheet.
5. Sprinkle with vegan cheese, if using.
6. Bake for 15-20 minutes, until peppers are tender.
7. Serve warm.

13. Baked Kale Chips

Ingredients:

- 1 bunch kale, stems removed and leaves torn into bite-sized pieces
- 1 tablespoon olive oil
- 1/4 teaspoon salt
- 1/4 teaspoon garlic powder
- 1/4 teaspoon paprika

Instructions:
1. Preheat the oven to 300°F (150°C).
2. In a bowl, toss kale leaves with olive oil, salt, garlic powder, and paprika.
3. Spread kale in a single layer on a baking sheet.
4. Bake for 10-15 minutes, until crisp.
5. Let cool before serving.

14. Avocado and Tomato Salad

Ingredients:
- 1 avocado, diced
- 1 tomato, diced
- 1/4 cup red onion, diced
- 2 tablespoons lime juice
- 1 tablespoon olive oil
- 1 tablespoon cilantro, chopped
- 1/4 teaspoon salt
- 1/4 teaspoon black pepper

Instructions:
1. In a bowl, combine avocado, tomato, red onion, lime juice, olive oil, cilantro, salt, and black pepper.
2. Toss gently to combine.
3. Serve chilled.

15. Rice Paper Spring Rolls

Ingredients:
- 8 rice paper wrappers

- 2 cups mixed greens
- 1 carrot, julienned
- 1 cucumber, julienned
- 1/2 bell pepper, julienned
- Fresh mint leaves
- Peanut sauce for dipping

Instructions:
1. Dip a rice paper wrapper in warm water for a few seconds to soften.
2. Place a handful of mixed greens on the bottom third of the wrapper.
3. Top with carrot, cucumber, bell pepper, and mint leaves.
4. Fold the bottom of the wrapper over the filling, then fold in the sides, and roll up tightly.
5. Repeat with remaining wrappers and filling.
6. Serve with peanut sauce for dipping.

16. Roasted Brussels Sprouts

Ingredients:
- 1 pound Brussels sprouts, halved
- 1 tablespoon olive oil
- 1/4 teaspoon salt
- 1/4 teaspoon black pepper
- 1/4 teaspoon garlic powder

Instructions:
1. Preheat the oven to 400°F (200°C).
2. Toss Brussels sprouts with olive oil, salt, black pepper, and garlic powder.
3. Spread Brussels sprouts in a single layer on a baking sheet.
4. Roast for 20-25 minutes, until tender and caramelized.
5. Serve warm.

17. Beet and Orange Salad

Ingredients:

- 2 beets, roasted, peeled, and diced
- 2 oranges, peeled and segmented
- 1/4 cup red onion, thinly sliced
- 2 tablespoons balsamic vinegar
- 1 tablespoon olive oil
- 1 tablespoon honey
- 1/4 teaspoon black pepper
- Fresh parsley, chopped for garnish

Instructions:
1. In a bowl, combine diced beets, orange segments, and red onion.
2. In a separate bowl, whisk together balsamic vinegar, olive oil, honey, and black pepper.
3. Pour dressing over beet mixture and toss to coat.
4. Sprinkle with chopped parsley before serving.

18. Roasted Red Pepper Hummus

Ingredients:
- 1 can chickpeas, drained and rinsed
- 1 roasted red pepper, peeled and chopped
- 2 tablespoons tahini
- 2 tablespoons lemon juice
- 1 garlic clove, minced
- 1/4 teaspoon cumin
- 1/4 teaspoon paprika
- Carrot, cucumber, and bell pepper sticks for dipping

Instructions:
1. In a food processor, combine chickpeas, roasted red pepper, tahini, lemon juice, garlic, cumin, and paprika.
2. Blend until smooth.
3. Serve with veggie sticks for dipping.

19. Spinach and Artichoke Dip

Ingredients:
- 1 can artichoke hearts, drained and chopped
- 1 cup frozen spinach, thawed and drained
- 1/2 cup Greek yogurt
- 1/4 cup mayonnaise
- 1/4 cup grated Parmesan cheese
- 1/4 cup grated mozzarella cheese
- 1 garlic clove, minced
- 1/4 teaspoon black pepper

Instructions:
1. Preheat the oven to 350°F (175°C).
2. In a bowl, combine chopped artichoke hearts, thawed spinach, Greek yogurt, mayonnaise, Parmesan cheese, mozzarella cheese, garlic, and black pepper.
3. Transfer mixture to a baking dish.
4. Bake for 25-30 minutes, until bubbly and golden brown on top.
5. Serve warm with whole grain crackers or veggie sticks.

20. Mixed Berry Smoothie

Ingredients:
- 1 cup mixed berries (strawberries, blueberries, raspberries)
- 1 banana
- 1 cup spinach leaves
- 1 cup almond milk
- 1 tablespoon chia seeds
- 1 tablespoon honey

Instructions:
1. Blend mixed berries, banana, spinach, almond milk, chia seeds, and honey until smooth.
2. Serve immediately.

Chapter 6: Desserts

1. Chia Seed Pudding

Ingredients:
- 1/4 cup chia seeds
- 1 cup almond milk
- 1 tablespoon honey
- 1/2 teaspoon vanilla extract
- Fresh berries for topping

Instructions:
1. In a bowl, mix chia seeds, almond milk, honey, and vanilla extract.
2. Cover and refrigerate for at least 2 hours, or overnight, until thickened.
3. Serve topped with fresh berries.

2. Baked Apples

Ingredients:
- 2 apples, cored
- 2 tablespoons oats
- 1 tablespoon chopped almonds
- 1 tablespoon raisins
- 1/2 teaspoon cinnamon
- 1/2 teaspoon nutmeg
- 1/2 cup water

Instructions:
1. Preheat the oven to 375°F (190°C).
2. In a bowl, mix oats, chopped almonds, raisins, cinnamon, and nutmeg.
3. Stuff each apple with the oat mixture.
4. Place stuffed apples in a baking dish and pour water into the bottom of the dish.
5. Bake for 30-40 minutes, until the apples are tender.
6. Serve warm.

3. Banana Ice Cream

Ingredients:
- 2 ripe bananas, sliced and frozen
- 1 tablespoon cocoa powder
- 1/2 teaspoon vanilla extract
- 2 tablespoons almond milk
- Chopped nuts for topping (optional)

Instructions:
1. Blend frozen banana slices, cocoa powder, vanilla extract, and almond milk in a blender until smooth.
2. Serve immediately, topped with chopped nuts if desired.

4. Berry Parfait

Ingredients:
- 1 cup mixed berries (strawberries, blueberries, raspberries)
- 1 cup Greek yogurt
- 2 tablespoons honey
- 1/4 cup granola

Instructions:
1. In a glass, layer mixed berries, Greek yogurt, honey, and granola.
2. Repeat layers.
3. Serve chilled.

5. Rice Pudding

Ingredients:
- 1/2 cup white rice
- 2 cups almond milk
- 1/4 cup honey
- 1/2 teaspoon cinnamon

- 1/2 teaspoon vanilla extract
- 1/4 cup raisins (optional)

Instructions:
1. In a saucepan, combine rice and almond milk.
2. Bring to a boil, then reduce heat and simmer for 20-25 minutes, stirring occasionally, until rice is tender and mixture is creamy.
3. Stir in honey, cinnamon, vanilla extract, and raisins, if using.
4. Cook for another 5 minutes.
5. Serve warm or chilled.

6. Oatmeal Cookies

Ingredients:
- 1 cup oats
- 1/2 cup whole wheat flour
- 1/4 cup honey
- 1/4 cup coconut oil, melted
- 1/2 teaspoon baking soda
- 1/2 teaspoon cinnamon
- 1/4 teaspoon salt
- 1/4 cup raisins

Instructions:
1. Preheat the oven to 350°F (175°C).
2. In a bowl, mix oats, whole wheat flour, honey, coconut oil, baking soda, cinnamon, salt, and raisins.
3. Drop spoonfuls of dough onto a baking sheet lined with parchment paper.
4. Flatten each cookie with a fork.
5. Bake for 10-12 minutes, until golden brown.
6. Let cool before serving.

7. Coconut Mango Sorbet

Ingredients:
- 2 cups frozen mango chunks
- 1/2 cup coconut milk
- 1 tablespoon lime juice
- 2 tablespoons shredded coconut for topping

Instructions:
1. Blend frozen mango chunks, coconut milk, and lime juice in a blender until smooth.
2. Serve immediately, topped with shredded coconut.

8. Peanut Butter Banana Bites

Ingredients:
- 1 banana, sliced
- 2 tablespoons peanut butter
- 2 tablespoons granola

Instructions:
1. Spread peanut butter on banana slices.
2. Sprinkle granola on top.
3. Serve immediately.

9. Chocolate Avocado Mousse

Ingredients:
- 1 ripe avocado
- 2 tablespoons cocoa powder
- 2 tablespoons honey
- 1/2 teaspoon vanilla extract
- 2 tablespoons almond milk

Instructions:
1. Blend avocado, cocoa powder, honey, vanilla extract, and almond milk in a blender until smooth.

2. Serve chilled.

10. Almond Joy Energy Bites

Ingredients:
- 1/2 cup almonds
- 1/2 cup dates, pitted
- 2 tablespoons cocoa powder
- 1/2 teaspoon vanilla extract
- 1/4 cup shredded coconut

Instructions:
1. Blend almonds, dates, cocoa powder, and vanilla extract in a food processor until mixture sticks together.
2. Roll mixture into small balls.
3. Roll balls in shredded coconut.
4. Serve chilled.

11. Apple Crisp

Ingredients:
- 4 apples, peeled and sliced
- 1/2 cup oats
- 1/4 cup almond flour
- 1/4 cup chopped almonds
- 2 tablespoons honey
- 1/2 teaspoon cinnamon
- 1/4 teaspoon nutmeg
- 2 tablespoons coconut oil, melted

Instructions:
1. Preheat the oven to 350°F (175°C).
2. Place apple slices in a baking dish.
3. In a bowl, combine oats, almond flour, chopped almonds, honey, cinnamon, nutmeg, and melted coconut oil.

4. Sprinkle oat mixture over apples.
5. Bake for 30-35 minutes, until the apples are tender and the topping is golden brown.
6. Serve warm.

12. Banana Bread

Ingredients:
- 2 ripe bananas, mashed
- 1/4 cup honey
- 1/4 cup coconut oil, melted
- 1/2 teaspoon vanilla extract
- 1/2 cup almond flour
- 1/2 cup oat flour
- 1/2 teaspoon baking soda
- 1/2 teaspoon cinnamon
- 1/4 teaspoon salt

Instructions:
1. Preheat the oven to 350°F (175°C).
2. In a bowl, mix mashed bananas, honey, coconut oil, and vanilla extract.
3. Add almond flour, oat flour, baking soda, cinnamon, and salt. Stir until combined.
4. Pour batter into a greased loaf pan.
5. Bake for 45-50 minutes, until a toothpick inserted into the center comes out clean.
6. Let cool before slicing.

13. Berry Crumble

Ingredients:
- 2 cups mixed berries (strawberries, blueberries, raspberries)
- 1/4 cup almond flour
- 1/4 cup oats
- 2 tablespoons chopped almonds

- 2 tablespoons honey
- 1/2 teaspoon cinnamon
- 2 tablespoons coconut oil, melted

Instructions:
1. Preheat the oven to 350°F (175°C).
2. In a bowl, mix mixed berries with almond flour, oats, chopped almonds, honey, and cinnamon.
3. Transfer berry mixture to a baking dish.
4. In the same bowl, mix melted coconut oil with a little more almond flour, oats, chopped almonds, honey, and cinnamon to create a crumbly topping.
5. Sprinkle crumble topping over the berry mixture.
6. Bake for 25-30 minutes, until the topping is golden brown and the berries are bubbly.
7. Serve warm.

14. Peach Sorbet

Ingredients:
- 2 cups frozen peach slices
- 1/2 cup coconut milk
- 1 tablespoon honey
- 1/2 teaspoon vanilla extract

Instructions:
1. Blend frozen peach slices, coconut milk, honey, and vanilla extract in a blender until smooth.
2. Serve immediately.

15. Lemon Poppy Seed Muffins

Ingredients:
- 1/2 cup almond flour
- 1/2 cup oat flour
- 1/4 cup honey

- 1/4 cup coconut oil, melted
- 1/4 cup almond milk
- 1 egg
- 1 tablespoon lemon zest
- 1 tablespoon lemon juice
- 1 tablespoon poppy seeds
- 1/2 teaspoon baking soda
- 1/4 teaspoon salt

Instructions:
1. Preheat the oven to 350°F (175°C).
2. In a bowl, mix almond flour, oat flour, honey, coconut oil, almond milk, egg, lemon zest, lemon juice, poppy seeds, baking soda, and salt.
3. Pour batter into muffin cups.
4. Bake for 20-25 minutes, until a toothpick inserted into the center comes out clean.
5. Let cool before serving.

16. Pumpkin Spice Energy Balls

Ingredients:
- 1/2 cup pumpkin puree
- 1/4 cup almond butter
- 2 tablespoons honey
- 1/2 teaspoon vanilla extract
- 1/2 teaspoon cinnamon
- 1/4 teaspoon nutmeg
- 1/4 teaspoon ginger
- 1/4 cup oats
- 1/4 cup almond flour

Instructions:
1. In a bowl, mix pumpkin puree, almond butter, honey, vanilla extract, cinnamon, nutmeg, and ginger.
2. Stir in oats and almond flour until well combined.

3. Roll mixture into balls.
4. Refrigerate for at least 30 minutes before serving.

17. Chocolate Covered Strawberries

Ingredients:
- 1/2 cup dark chocolate chips
- 10 strawberries, washed and dried

Instructions:
1. Melt dark chocolate chips in a microwave-safe bowl in 30-second intervals, stirring in between, until smooth.
2. Dip strawberries into melted chocolate, covering about half of each strawberry.
3. Place strawberries on a parchment-lined baking sheet.
4. Refrigerate for 30 minutes, until chocolate is set.
5. Serve chilled.

18. Mango Sticky Rice

Ingredients:
- 1 cup sticky rice, cooked
- 1 ripe mango, sliced
- 1/2 cup coconut milk
- 2 tablespoons honey
- Toasted sesame seeds for topping

Instructions:
1. In a bowl, mix cooked sticky rice with coconut milk and honey.
2. Serve sticky rice with sliced mango on top.
3. Sprinkle it with toasted sesame seeds.

19. Blueberry Lemon Sorbet

Ingredients:

- 2 cups frozen blueberries
- 1/4 cup honey
- 1/4 cup lemon juice
- 1/2 teaspoon lemon zest

Instructions:
1. Blend frozen blueberries, honey, lemon juice, and lemon zest in a blender until smooth.
2. Serve immediately.

20. Pistachio Date Balls

Ingredients:
- 1/2 cup pistachios
- 1/2 cup dates, pitted
- 1/4 cup shredded coconut

Instructions:
1. Blend pistachios and dates in a food processor until mixture sticks together.
2. Roll mixture into balls.
3. Roll balls in shredded coconut.
4. Serve chilled.

Chapter 7: Drinks and Smoothies

1. Green Smoothie

Ingredients:
- 1 cup spinach
- 1/2 cup cucumber, chopped
- 1/2 banana
- 1/2 cup almond milk
- 1/2 cup water
- 1 tablespoon chia seeds
- 1 tablespoon honey

Instructions:
1. Blend spinach, cucumber, banana, almond milk, water, chia seeds, and honey until smooth.
2. Serve immediately.

2. Berry Blast Smoothie

Ingredients:
- 1/2 cup mixed berries (strawberries, blueberries, raspberries)
- 1/2 banana
- 1/2 cup almond milk
- 1/2 cup water
- 1 tablespoon flax seeds
- 1 tablespoon honey

Instructions:
1. Blend mixed berries, banana, almond milk, water, flaxseeds, and honey until smooth.
2. Serve immediately.

3. Golden Milk

Ingredients:
- 1 cup almond milk
- 1 teaspoon turmeric
- 1/2 teaspoon cinnamon
- 1/4 teaspoon ginger
- 1/4 teaspoon cardamom
- 1 tablespoon honey

Instructions:
1. Heat almond milk in a saucepan over medium heat.
2. Stir in turmeric, cinnamon, ginger, cardamom, and honey until well combined.
3. Serve warm.

4. Watermelon Cooler

Ingredients:
- 2 cups watermelon, cubed
- 1/2 cup coconut water
- 1 tablespoon lime juice
- Mint leaves for garnish

Instructions:
1. Blend watermelon, coconut water, and lime juice until smooth.
2. Serve chilled, garnished with mint leaves.

5. Cucumber Mint Infused Water

Ingredients:
- 8 cups water
- 1 cucumber, thinly sliced
- 1/4 cup fresh mint leaves

Instructions:
1. Combine water, cucumber slices, and mint leaves in a pitcher.

2. Refrigerate for at least 2 hours, or overnight, before serving.

6. Herbal Tea

Ingredients:
- 1 herbal tea bag (such as chamomile or peppermint)
- 1 cup hot water
- 1 tablespoon honey

Instructions:
1. Steep herbal tea bags in hot water for 3-5 minutes.
2. Stir in honey until dissolved.
3. Serve warm.

7. Carrot Ginger Juice

Ingredients:
- 2 carrots, chopped
- 1/2 inch ginger, peeled
- 1/2 cup water
- 1 tablespoon lemon juice

Instructions:
1. Blend carrots, ginger, water, and lemon juice until smooth.
2. Strain juice through a fine mesh sieve.
3. Serve chilled.

8. Pineapple Coconut Smoothie

Ingredients:
- 1 cup pineapple chunks
- 1/2 banana
- 1/2 cup coconut milk
- 1/2 cup water
- 1 tablespoon shredded coconut

Instructions:
1. Blend pineapple chunks, banana, coconut milk, water, and shredded coconut until smooth.
2. Serve immediately.

9. Beetroot and Berry Juice

Ingredients:
- 1 small beetroot, peeled and chopped
- 1/2 cup mixed berries (strawberries, blueberries, raspberries)
- 1/2 cup water
- 1 tablespoon honey

Instructions:
1. Blend beetroot, mixed berries, water, and honey until smooth.
2. Strain juice through a fine mesh sieve.
3. Serve chilled.

10. Almond Butter Banana Smoothie

Ingredients:
- 1 banana
- 1 tablespoon almond butter
- 1/2 cup almond milk
- 1/2 cup water
- 1 tablespoon chia seeds

Instructions:
1. Blend banana, almond butter, almond milk, water, and chia seeds until smooth.
2. Serve immediately.

11. Avocado Spinach Smoothie

Ingredients:
- 1/2 avocado
- 1 cup spinach
- 1/2 banana
- 1/2 cup almond milk
- 1/2 cup water
- 1 tablespoon honey

Instructions:
1. Blend avocado, spinach, banana, almond milk, water, and honey until smooth.
2. Serve immediately.

12. Tomato Basil Infused Water

Ingredients:
- 8 cups water
- 1 cup cherry tomatoes, halved
- 1/4 cup fresh basil leaves

Instructions:
1. Combine water, cherry tomatoes, and basil leaves in a pitcher.
2. Refrigerate for at least 2 hours, or overnight, before serving.

13. Berry Green Tea

Ingredients:
- 1 green tea bag
- 1 cup hot water
- 1/2 cup mixed berries (strawberries, blueberries, raspberries)
- 1 tablespoon honey

Instructions:
1. Steep green tea bags in hot water for 3-5 minutes.
2. Remove the tea bag and stir in mixed berries and honey.

3. Serve warm or chilled.

14. Mango Lassi

Ingredients:
- 1 cup mango chunks
- 1/2 cup Greek yogurt
- 1/2 cup almond milk
- 1/2 cup water
- 1 tablespoon honey
- 1/4 teaspoon cardamom

Instructions:
1. Blend mango chunks, Greek yogurt, almond milk, water, honey, and cardamom until smooth.
2. Serve chilled.

15. Lemon Ginger Detox Water

Ingredients:
- 8 cups water
- 1 lemon, thinly sliced
- 1 inch ginger, peeled and thinly sliced

Instructions:
1. Combine water, lemon slices, and ginger slices in a pitcher.
2. Refrigerate for at least 2 hours, or overnight, before serving.

16. Peach Basil Iced Tea

Ingredients:
- 4 cups water
- 4 black tea bags
- 2 peaches, pitted and sliced
- 1/4 cup fresh basil leaves

- 2 tablespoons honey

Instructions:
1. Bring water to a boil in a saucepan.
2. Remove from heat and add tea bags. Steep for 5 minutes.
3. Remove tea bags and let tea cool to room temperature.
4. Blend peaches, basil leaves, and honey until smooth.
5. Strain peach mixture through a fine mesh sieve into the tea.
6. Serve over ice.

17. Orange Carrot Ginger Juice

Ingredients:
- 2 oranges, peeled
- 2 carrots, chopped
- 1/2 inch ginger, peeled
- 1/2 cup water

Instructions:
1. Blend oranges, carrots, ginger, and water until smooth.
2. Strain juice through a fine mesh sieve.
3. Serve chilled.

18. Raspberry Coconut Smoothie

Ingredients:
- 1/2 cup raspberries
- 1/2 banana
- 1/2 cup coconut milk
- 1/2 cup water
- 1 tablespoon chia seeds

Instructions:
1. Blend raspberries, banana, coconut milk, water, and chia seeds until smooth.

2. Serve immediately.

19. Pineapple Mint Infused Water

Ingredients:
- 8 cups water
- 1 cup pineapple chunks
- 1/4 cup fresh mint leaves

Instructions:
1. Combine water, pineapple chunks, and mint leaves in a pitcher.
2. Refrigerate for at least 2 hours, or overnight, before serving.

20. Blueberry Almond Smoothie

Ingredients:
- 1/2 cup blueberries
- 1/2 banana
- 1/2 cup almond milk
- 1/2 cup water
- 1 tablespoon almond butter

Instructions:
1. Blend blueberries, banana, almond milk, water, and almond butter until smooth.
2. Serve immediately.

Chapter 8: Supplements and Nutrition

- Important Supplements for Vegetarians with Kidney Disease

People with kidney disease, especially those following a vegetarian diet, may benefit from certain supplements to ensure they are meeting their nutritional needs. Here are some important supplements to consider:

1. Vitamin B12

- Why it's important: Vitamin B12 is primarily found in animal products and is essential for nerve function and red blood cell production.
- Supplement form: Cyanocobalamin or methylcobalamin.
- Dosage: Consult a healthcare provider for the appropriate dosage, as individual needs vary.

2. Iron

- Why it's important: Iron deficiency can lead to anemia, especially in people with kidney disease who may already have lower red blood cell counts.
- Supplement form: Ferrous sulfate or ferrous gluconate.
- Dosage: Consult a healthcare provider for the appropriate dosage, as too much iron can be harmful.

3. Vitamin D

- Why it's important: Vitamin D helps maintain bone health and may play a role in kidney disease management.
- Supplement form: Vitamin D3 (cholecalciferol).
- Dosage: Consult a healthcare provider for the appropriate dosage, as too much vitamin D can be harmful.

4. Omega-3 Fatty Acids

- Why they're important: Omega-3s have anti-inflammatory properties and may benefit kidney health.
- Supplement form: Fish oil or algae-based supplements.
- Dosage: Consult a healthcare provider for the appropriate dosage.

5. Calcium

- Why it's important: Calcium is important for bone health, but people with kidney disease need to be cautious about calcium supplements due to the risk of hypercalcemia.
- Supplement form: Calcium citrate.
- Dosage: Consult a healthcare provider for the appropriate dosage and monitoring.

6. Phosphorus Binders

- Why they're important: Phosphorus control is crucial for kidney disease management, and phosphorus binders can help reduce phosphorus absorption from food.
- Supplement form: Available by prescription.
- Dosage: Follow the prescribed dosage and instructions from your healthcare provider.

7. Multivitamin

- Why it's important: A well-formulated multivitamin can help fill gaps in essential nutrients for vegetarians with kidney disease.
- Supplement form: Choose a multivitamin specifically designed for people with kidney disease.
- Dosage: Follow the recommended dosage on the label or as advised by a healthcare provider.

Always consult with a healthcare provider before starting any new supplements, as they can interact with medications and affect kidney function. Regular monitoring of nutrient levels is important for individuals with kidney disease to prevent deficiencies and maintain overall health.

- How to Talk to Your Doctor About Supplement

When discussing supplements with your doctor, it's important to communicate openly and effectively to ensure you receive the best advice and guidance. Here are some tips on how to talk to your doctor about supplements:

1. Prepare in Advance: Make a list of all the supplements you are currently taking, including the dosage and frequency. Also, jot down any specific questions or concerns you have about supplements.

2. Be Honest: Provide your doctor with accurate information about your supplement use, including any herbal remedies or vitamins you may be taking. This will help your doctor understand your overall health and make informed recommendations.

3. Ask Questions: Don't hesitate to ask questions about supplements, including their benefits, potential side effects, and interactions with other medications you may be taking.

4. Discuss Your Goals: Explain why you are taking or considering taking supplements and what you hope to achieve. Your doctor can help you determine if supplements are the right choice for you and if there are alternative options.

5. Consider Medical History: Share any relevant medical history, including kidney disease, allergies, or other conditions, as this can impact the safety and effectiveness of supplements.

6. Follow Your Doctor's Recommendations: Based on your discussion, your doctor may recommend specific supplements, adjust your current regimen, or advise against certain supplements. Follow their advice carefully.

7. Monitor Your Health: After starting or changing supplements, pay attention to how your body responds. If you experience any adverse effects, contact your doctor immediately.

8. Regular Follow-Up: Schedule regular check-ups with your doctor to monitor your health and discuss any changes in your supplement regimen or health status.

By having an open and honest conversation with your doctor, you can work together to ensure that any supplements you take are safe, effective, and beneficial for your health.

- Managing Protein Intake

Managing protein intake is crucial for individuals with kidney disease, especially those following a vegetarian diet. Here are some tips for managing protein intake:

1. Choose High-Quality Proteins: Opt for high-quality protein sources that are low in phosphorus and potassium, such as egg whites, tofu, and tempeh.

2. Limit Phosphorus: Some plant-based protein sources, like beans and lentils, are high in phosphorus. To lower phosphorus intake, soak beans before cooking and choose lower-phosphorus options more often, such as tofu or tempeh.

3. Control Portion Sizes: Be mindful of portion sizes to avoid consuming too much protein. Use measuring cups or a food scale to accurately measure portions.

4. Balance Protein with Carbohydrates: Pairing protein-rich foods with carbohydrates can help reduce the amount of protein your body needs to break down, easing the burden on your kidneys. For example, enjoy beans with rice or tofu with quinoa.

5. Monitor Protein Intake: Keep track of your daily protein intake to ensure you are meeting your needs without exceeding them. A dietitian can help you determine your specific protein requirements.

6. Consider Protein Supplements: In some cases, protein supplements may be necessary to meet protein needs. However, it's essential to choose supplements that are low in phosphorus and potassium.

7. Consult a Dietitian: A registered dietitian can help you create a personalized meal plan that meets your protein needs while considering your kidney health and dietary preferences.

8. Stay Hydrated: Drinking plenty of water can help flush out waste products from protein metabolism and reduce the strain on your kidneys.

By managing your protein intake carefully and making smart food choices, you can help protect your kidney health and overall well-being.

Chapter 9: 7-Day Meal Plan

Day 1

Breakfast:
- Spinach and Mushroom Omelette
- Whole Grain Toast
- Cucumber Mint Infused Water

Lunch:
- Avocado Spinach Smoothie
- Mixed Berry Parfait with Greek Yogurt and Granola

Dinner:
- Lentil and Sweet Potato Curry with Brown Rice
- Side Salad with Lemon Vinaigrette

Dessert:
- Apple Crisp with Almond Crumble
- Herbal Tea

Snack:
- Carrot Sticks with Hummus
- Almonds

Day 2

Breakfast:
- Berry Blast Smoothie
- Whole Grain Pancakes with Maple Syrup

Lunch:
- Chickpea Salad with Lemon Tahini Dressing
- Whole Grain Pita Bread

Dinner:
- Vegetable Stir-Fry with Tofu and Quinoa
- Steamed Edamame

Dessert:
- Banana Bread Slices
- Chamomile Tea

Snack:
- Almond Butter on Rice Cakes
- Fresh Berries

Day 3

Breakfast:
- Golden Milk
- Oatmeal with Sliced Almonds and Honey

Lunch:
- Mediterranean Quinoa Salad
- Whole Grain Crackers

Dinner:
- Stuffed Bell Peppers with Tomato Basil Sauce
- Roasted Asparagus

Dessert:
- Berry Crumble with Greek Yogurt
- Rooibos Tea

Snack:
- Greek Yogurt with Honey and Walnuts
- Apple Slices

Day 4

Breakfast:
- Orange Carrot Ginger Juice
- Whole Grain Waffles with Fresh Berries

Lunch:
- Lentil Soup with Whole Grain Bread
- Side Salad with Balsamic Dressing

Dinner:
- Spinach and Mushroom Stuffed Portobello Mushrooms
- Quinoa Salad

Dessert:
- Mango Sticky Rice
- Green Tea

Snack:
- Rice Cakes with Almond Butter
- Celery Sticks

Day 5

Breakfast:
- Berry Green Tea Smoothie
- Avocado Toast on Whole Grain Bread

Lunch:
- Quinoa Black Bean Salad
- Whole Grain Tortilla Chips

Dinner:
- Vegetable Curry with Coconut Milk and Basmati Rice
- Steamed Broccoli

Dessert:
- Peach Basil Iced Tea
- Coconut Macaroons

Snack:
- Mixed Nuts
- Fresh Fruit Salad

Day 6

Breakfast:
- Lemon Ginger Detox Water
- Greek Yogurt Parfait with Granola and Mixed Berries

Lunch:
- Sweet Potato and Black Bean Tacos
- Mexican Street Corn

Dinner:
- Mushroom Risotto with Asparagus
- Side Salad with Citrus Dressing

Dessert:
- Blueberry Lemon Sorbet
- Sparkling Water with Lemon

Snack:
- Pumpkin Seeds
- Cherry Tomatoes with Mozzarella

Day 7

Breakfast:
- Pineapple Mint Infused Water
- Whole Grain Bagel with Cream Cheese and Sliced Tomato

Lunch:
- Lentil Spinach Soup with Whole Grain Bread
- Caprese Salad

Dinner:
- Ratatouille with Herbed Quinoa
- Garlic Bread

Dessert:
- Pistachio Date Balls
- Iced Herbal Tea

Snack:
- Celery Sticks with Peanut Butter
- Dried Fruit Mix

- **Shopping List for the Week**

Produce:
- Spinach
- Mushrooms
- Eggs
- Avocado
- Sweet potatoes
- Apples
- Lemons
- Berries (strawberries, blueberries, raspberries)
- Bananas
- Cucumber
- Mint leaves
- Cherry tomatoes
- Basil
- Ginger
- Carrots
- Oranges
- Peaches
- Asparagus
- Bell peppers
- Tomato
- Broccoli
- Edamame
- Green beans
- Garlic
- Onion
- Zucchini
- Eggplant
- Corn
- Pineapple
- Celery
- Tomato
- Fresh herbs (optional)

Dairy/Non-Dairy:
- Greek yogurt
- Almond milk
- Coconut milk
- Cream cheese
- Mozzarella cheese
- Butter

Grains/Carbs:
- Whole grain bread
- Whole grain tortilla chips
- Whole grain crackers
- Whole grain pasta
- Brown rice
- Quinoa
- Oatmeal
- Whole grain waffles
- Whole grain pancake mix
- Whole grain bagels
- Granola
- Rice cakes
- Whole grain tortillas

Proteins:
- Tofu
- Tempeh
- Lentils
- Chickpeas
- Black beans
- Almonds
- Almond butter
- Peanut butter

Frozen:
- Mixed berries

- Mango chunks
- Spinach
- Corn

Pantry Staples:
- Olive oil
- Coconut oil
- Honey
- Maple syrup
- Chia seeds
- Flaxseeds
- Almond flour
- Baking powder
- Baking soda
- Cinnamon
- Vanilla extract
- Turmeric
- Cardamom
- Cumin
- Coriander
- Paprika
- Nutritional yeast
- Vegetable broth

Snacks/Desserts:
- Hummus
- Granola bars
- Dark chocolate
- Rice cakes
- Mixed nuts
- Coconut macaroons
- Dried fruit mix
- Popcorn kernels

Beverages:

- Herbal tea (chamomile, rooibos)
- Sparkling water

This list may vary based on your pantry staples and personal preferences. Adjust quantities based on the number of servings needed for your meals.

Conclusion

As you embark on this journey to nourish your body and support your kidney health with wholesome, plant-based meals, remember to be kind to yourself. Change takes time, and every step you take towards a healthier lifestyle is a step in the right direction. Embrace the process, listen to your body, and savor the flavors and textures of each meal. Your health and well-being are worth the effort, and with each meal, you are nurturing not just your body, but also your spirit. Here's to your health and happiness, one delicious meal at a time.

Printed in Great Britain
by Amazon